My Health and Fitness

I0429482

Volume 4

52 Articles

By: Wade Yoder

Master Trainer - Fitness Nutrition Specialist

- Health & Fitness Columnist

I would like to dedicate this volume to the special people in my life.

My Dad: as far back as I can remember he studied nutrition, exercised and has stayed consistent with it throughout his life. My dad always exercised at home so it didn't take time away from being with us. He is 76 years old, working full time (much of what is physically intensive) and still enjoys his exercise sessions. His approach to life, family and the way he treats people has always been a good example to me and there is no man on the planet that I admire more than my Dad. Thanks Pop, you are my hero!

My Mom: my Mom raised 8 children, was a professional caterer for 25 years and is the author of 3 cookbooks. She did all this while at the same time keeping balance in the home and keeping her children healthy. She has shown me how powerful the work can be of a person that is willing to work behind the scenes and how oft times it's the unglamorous steady work behind the scenes that yields great results. My mom reminds me of a passage of scripture in Proverbs that says, "A virtuous women's price is far more precious than rubies." I was and am lucky to have her as my Mom and the combination of her and my dad as parents of our family was and is a blessing beyond measure- Love you Mom

My uncle Richard: (my mom's twin brother) is a big inspiration to me. He is a medical doctor and his passion for healing and for helping hurting people both domestically and in foreign countries has set an example to me as well. He serves more on the intervention side of healthcare and mine is in prevention so there are some things we don't always agree on but he helps me keep a more balanced perspective in the progression of medicine and prevention. Thanks uncle Richard

My son and daughter: my son and daughter are life's best gifts to me and make me want to do better as well as do my part in helping to make the world a better place. Love you Nicole and Caleb

Newspapers: I want to thank the newspapers that have been publishing my articles (Leader Tribune, Citizen Georgian, Taylor County News, Georgia Post and The News Observer) it's an honor to be your health and fitness columnist.

There are far too many people to list here, but to my family, friends, members of my health club, my readers, community and surrounding communities, I would like to thank you for being the inspiration for these articles and books. You are my reasons why~ Wade Yoder

About the author

Wade Yoder has been in the health and fitness club business since 1991 and is a weekly health and fitness columnist for 5 Middle, Georgia newspapers with over 200 published articles since 2012.
He owns and operates Valley Athletic Club in Fort Valley, Georgia

Master Trainer certifications:

Fitness Trainer - Fitness Nutrition

Fitness Therapy - Strength and Conditioning

Senior Fitness & Youth Fitness

Legal Disclaimer: many of these articles have been written using the author's opinion on things that have been drawn from over 20 years of experience in health, fitness and nutrition, and as a health club operator since 1991, (please use this information as such). If you use information and advice in this volume of articles, you agree to hold the author harmless.

Table of Contents

To Attempt to Live Longer is Nuts!

Some research recently caught my attention and nutty as it may have sounded, the research showed that death from the leading causes (heart disease, cancer, and respiratory), were lower in ones with higher nut consumption. This research from Brigham and Women's Hospital, and Harvard Medical School looked at nut consumption and deaths from all causes among 76,464 women participating in the Nurse's Health Study and 42,498 men involved in the Health Professionals Follow-up Study.

The nuts in this study were: almonds, cashews, hazelnuts, macadamias, pecans, pine nuts, pistachios and walnuts.

One thing I really liked about this research was, though partially funded by the International Tree Nut Council Nutrition Research & Education Foundation, (a non-profit organization representing nine tree nut industries) they had no role in the research or results. This is how all studies should be conducted.

What they found was, ones who ate nuts seven or more times per week had a 20% lower death rate after four years than individuals who did not eat nuts. The nut consumers also tended to be leaner, more physically active and non-smokers.

Nuts over all are known to have heart healthy fats and are loaded with protein and vitamins as well as antioxidants that are thought to be linked to a lower risk of heart disease, and heart disease is the number one killer in America!

A study released by the CDC on 12-17-2014 found that about 60 percent of Americans don't consume nuts on a daily basis and the FDA says the ideal consumption is an ounce-and-a-half, in their guidelines for reducing heart disease.

Research also seems to be showing positive results in protecting the brain from the cellular and cognitive dysfunction associated with the aging process and neurodegenerative diseases.

The nuts in this excerpt were: walnuts, almonds, pistachios, and pecans.

Eating a variety of nuts should give added benefit from the various nutritional strong points of the individual nuts, but eating the ones that are grown in your home area should be the best ones. Pecans do very well in my home area, so pecans would definitely be my number one choice. And though not considered a tree nut, the good ole Georgia peanut is also one that I like.

Keeping nuts around in areas you're most likely to eat snacks, can be a good way to get more nuts in your diet and can be a constant reminder of what you are trying to do vs. aimlessly snacking on whatever happens to be in the vicinity. This will not only give you the potential benefits listed above, but will also give you some very vital nutrients (proteins and fats) for your 2015 exercise and fitness goals!

Fitness Starting Points

There are many starting points in life and fitness is no exception. You are unique because no two people are like each other, so what may be good for one person may not necessarily work as well for you. In fitness and health, we should look for our weak points, and when we bring that up to par with our strong points, the whole package will look and feel better!

Example: if you work behind a desk and have a friend that is a waitress, and you both decide to start a fitness program together, in the beginning you may have a little difficulty keeping up with your friend. You should give yourself a little more time to catch up, since she has already been exercising somewhat at work and you have a sedentary job. Recognizing this can help you avoid injury as well as inflammatory joint and connective tissue problems.

Starting points need to be made at your weak point(s) and simply connected to the type of routine you select, whether in training or diet. Once you know the things you want or need improvement in, (whether it's losing weight, gaining muscle, shaping up, remedying or preventing chronic disease or to become healthier) you simply find the recipe with the ingredients that will yield the results you want. The same ingredients do not apply for a German Chocolate cake as it does for a pound cake! Once we get the components of our fitness routine together, it works like a designer prescription in giving us the desired outcome!

Here are a few starting points that work for what most of us want at the beginning of the year:

1. Gain muscle.

2. Lose body fat.

3. Increasing endurance.

4. Fighting chronic disease with our own immune system.

1. Losing body fat: inside our fat cells are calories. These calories are what make the fat cell get larger. Most of us need at least 1600 to 2400 calories to fuel our daily needs, (some may need more, some less, mostly depending on the activity levels of the person and the amount of muscle he or she has). When we drop the amount of calories we take in (with absolutely no sugar intake) our body will literally suck out calories from our fatty deposits. Keep in mind that in order for this to happen, we must be willing to let the sugar level drop low enough in the blood to trigger the release of fat for energy. SUGAR IS THE NUMBER ONE ENEMY OF FAT RELEASE! Do not drop calories super low for longer then 36-48 hours or you will go into a catabolic (muscle breakdown) state.

2. Gaining muscle and tone: making your muscles do things they're not used to doing forces them to adapt. They adapt by firming up, building up and toning up and giving us a better shape. Muscle does not care how it looks, only that it can handle the new stress better!

3. Increasing endurance: most times what causes an increase in cardiopulmonary activity is simply working muscle. Working muscle needs a lot of blood and oxygen, so when we get a lot of muscle's working at the same time, it forces our heart and lungs to work harder. You don't have to spend a lot of time on cardio machines or other strictly aerobic activity to do this, (you can do this in your strengthening, toning and building routine as well), by sticking with large muscle groups with very little rest. The large muscle groups are worked usually when you have 2 or more joints moving during an exercise (compound movements). If there are things you do in daily life that cause you to get winded, doing these things oftener will build endurance as well.

4. Fighting chronic disease: most chronic disease (heart disease, cancer, diabetes, etc.) is connected to a shortfall in lifestyle habits. Find the one(s) you're lacking in and strengthen those habit(s) and your body will oft times start cleaning up the chronic condition or disease like a garbage disposal and sanitation system.

5. Questions we need to ask ourselves to become proactive at staying healthy or regaining health are:

1. Is the air I breathe clean?

2. Are the fluids I drink free from additives and chemicals?

3. Am I eating a balanced and healthy diet (primarily made up with foods that were foods 500 years ago)?

4. Am I getting daily activity and exercise? Am I getting deep sleep?

5. Am I getting out in the sun? Sun in moderate doses is vitamin D therapy.

6. Am I de-stressing by doing some things I enjoy on a regular basis? Stress is something that can slowly kill us, if we do not have a way to release it.

7. Am I staying socially active, and keeping my brain challenged by new or complex things? To stay strong, the brain needs activity, and just like our body, a lack of activity can cause a weakening of our control center as well!

It does not matter where your starting point is, (when you do what it takes to strengthen them combined with consistency), you can turn your weaknesses into your strengths...

How to Detox for Prevention, Energy and Fitness!

Probably most of us have either detoxed before or thought about doing a detox especially after we were older and more concerned about the bad stuff that might be building up inside us. Detoxing can be a really good thing if done properly and can have a lot of health benefits as well as slimming our mid-section. It also can make you feel really good about the foundation you give to your health and fitness goals in a new year!

We have a lot going on around us that is hard to control and to do the things we need to do, makes it hard to live in a perfect bubble. We have environmental toxins floating around us from things such as air fresheners, cleaning chemicals, makeup, deodorants etc. and then food toxins and sludge buildup inside us from a modern diet with not nearly enough fiber to eliminate properly. I tend to get upset about some of the things we get exposed to with very little knowledge and research on long-term health effects, but I've come to the conclusion that our best bet is to build our own defenses and capabilities to fend off and eliminate these things.

When these toxins build up in our body, our need for medicine and other external assistance is going to go up because our own immune system's ability to protect us from illness and disease is getting handcuffed!

A detox lifestyle: we have a waste system that is constantly trying to move toxic things out of our body, and if we can do a few things regularly, it can pretty much keep us detoxed as we go. This mostly boils down to plenty of water, active lifestyle and diet.

1. Movement stimulates the lymphatic system and waste removal systems.

2. A good diet keeps the food moving along with plenty of fiber, as well as loads of antioxidants that help neutralize things that cause disease.

3. Adequate water helps flush toxins out.

Detoxing to catch up: if we have been slack on our diet, doing a detox once or twice a year can help get our detoxification systems caught back up and back on top of things, (this detox can be done by changing food for around 7 days to a mostly raw plant based diet). Add in some coconut oil or olive oil (every day) and this will help your body pass old fecal matter better. This will help remove excess waste from the midsection and colon as well as to detox the liver and kidneys, (it's like a system reset).

There are some very good detox kits around that really help in a systemic cleanse of the colon, liver and kidneys. My favorite detox program is the 7-Day Lee Haney System Cleanse. Most everyone enjoys the slenderizing effect it has on the midsection, but the most important reason should always be to get toxic residue out of our system and keep it from leeching back into our body from our colon.

One thing that is really important is high fiber during a detox period. When we detox, our body starts releasing the toxins its been storing (in our body tissue), into our waste removal systems and in order to keep them from reabsorbing into our system, we need to eat plenty of fiber to bind to the toxins. This will help ensure that the toxins released will get dragged out through our waste instead of getting reabsorbed. A high fiber raw food diet (fruits, vegetables, nuts, etc.) works on toxins like a Swiffer sweeper works on binding to dirt when it goes across linoleum or tile floor.

A few things that can help boost toxin removal are: exercises that work large muscle groups, such as squats, jumping jacks, and rebounding. Up and down movement really helps move our lymph fluid in the direction it's supposed to go. Skin brushing with upward motions can help the lymphatic system as well. Plenty of water, sweating and antioxidant rich diet are big factors during a detox and to help with our body's daily detoxing efforts.

Detoxing can make a person feel sluggish and sometimes give flu like symptoms, but when you come out of the detox period, the fog lifts and usually with it comes a lot more energy! If your energy gets really low during your detox, take one or two teaspoons of raw honey to boost energy levels.

Keeping our body toxin free, helps us to not only unleash the power of the immune system, but happens to slenderize the waist as well! Oft times a good detox can get rid of 7-12 pounds of waste!

Too Much Exercise Can Stop Up Your Drain Pipe!

Yep, there can be such a thing as too much exercise and it can fit quite well with the saying "too much of a good thing can become a bad thing."

Someone called me recently out of concern for a granddaughter that had started an exercise regimen and had run into some pretty severe health complications and had to be hospitalized. I pretty quickly recognized the symptoms as ones that matched a case I had heard about several years ago, about a new member at a gym here in Georgia.

Both cases could've really ended badly due to one thing they both had in common; there was too much protein breakdown in too short a time period! Muscle breakdown is what happens when muscle does something that it's not used to doing. This is the process it goes through to build, tone or become stronger, and this is a good thing, but once again, too much of a good thing can become a really bad thing.

Another thing both girls had in common was urine turned dark like the color of a dark soda (due to all the protein breakdown), and if there is too much of this, it can lead to renal (kidney) failure.

Example: imagine too much debris being washed toward a drain opening that has a filter in it, it wouldn't be long before water starts backing up and causing a mess!

A simple assessment can be made prior to beginning a fitness routine, and that is a person's level of comparable activity in the weeks and months prior to starting. One of the girls above was an insurance agent and probably had very low levels of physical activities compared to someone with a physically demanding job. Trainers should look out for this and make a difference in the routine they set up for someone, after all exercise routines are not a one size fits all kind of thing.

Example: a carpenter could handle a much more intense exercise routine then a banker in the beginning. A strenuous routine would cause a lot more protein breakdown for the banker then for the carpenter.

A doctor can run a test to measure the creatine kinase (CK) levels in the blood and if it shows up as CK-MM, it will show where the high levels of creatine kinase is coming from and in this case it's coming from muscle injury. My personal opinion is that the level of CK-MM they find in the blood will be a good indicator of the amount of protein found in the urine and this seems to be the part that triggers renal (kidney) failure.

The breakdown phase: when we make our muscles strain and handle a workload they're not used to handling, it causes little microfiber tears (injury) to our muscle, which causes protein breakdown. This is a good thing, but when this happens on a mass scale, it can cause too much protein breakdown and can simply overwhelm our fluid waste removal system. This can lead to fluid retention simply from kidney overload.

The building phase: when we have protein breakdown, our body takes protein from our diet and breaks it down into amino acids, (and uses it like patch paint for the muscles). This is the toning, building and strengthening process. Our body recognizes the strain our muscle just went through and its need to handle the workload better, so it builds the muscle fiber back a little more capable then before. Muscle does not care what it looks like, only that it can handle the newly imposed stress better.

So not only does our body tote new material from our diet to build new muscle, it also has to tote off residue from the worksite. Give it time to do its job properly, especially in the beginning, or your body may display a few "Temporarily Out of Order signs!"

Tip: eliminating sodas from your diet can lighten the load on your kidneys, especially if you use water instead, (and btw water helps flush residue out, not add to it). Using some organic, unfiltered cranberry juice or extract can help with kidney health as well.

Remember: a consistent routine is much better then a radical and unsustainable routine and will lead to much better results without the risk of injury.

 Building the kind of body, strength and tone you want, is like a construction site, and every good construction site needs to allow adequate waste removal time before the next work day, or trash will clutter the worksite, slowing down performance as well as effecting the quality of construction!

Cellular Regeneration...
You are Trillions!

Though we are one body, we are made up of a massive amount of cells, whether they be skin cells, heart cells, lung cells, bone cells, fat cells, muscle cells, liver cells, kidney cells, I'm sure you get the idea. Its estimated to be over 50 trillion cells in an adult person and when we think of the massive scale of operations that happens with our body every single day, for me its nothing short of a master design, by a Master Creator and is much more powerful in its capabilities then we oft times give our body's regeneration system credit for.

When we do the right things for our body, it helps these trillions of cells give birth to new generations of cells that can help our body get rid of and fend off chronic disease and premature aging. A good place to start is to get the old stuff out (by doing a colon, kidney and liver cleanse), so the toxins won't keep leeching back into the system. After we do that, we can give our cells a good clean start! Eating plenty of fiber rich foods helps maintain our waste disposal system.

Our body produces and replaces millions of cells per second, (that's probably a very conservative number) and a lot of the health of these new cells, depends on our dietary intake and environmental surroundings. Our nutritional intake has a huge impact on the health of our cells, as well as how they communicate and behave with each other.

Example: we make about 2 million red blood cells every second, the health of these cells are really important since they are what transport two life giving substances to our body parts, (oxygen and nutrients). Without these two, areas of our body (if not the whole body) can get diseased and begin to die.

It takes approximately 3 months: to have an entirely new blood supply with new red blood cells replacing the old ones and this new generation is made from the nutrition we choose to consume. A good diet with iron rich foods helps build good blood. Such as, dark green leafy vegetables, beets, eggs, red meat, chicken and organ meats. A diet rich in vegetables, fruits and nuts (especially locally grown ones), helps build strong blood as well.

It takes approximately 6 months: for our soft tissue (skeletal muscle, heart, lungs etc.) throughout our body to be replaced by a new supply of cells. We can help the construction of these new cells with a good diet and exercise. Since most of our soft tissue is constructed with protein material (protein and hormones are major components of the building cycle), so we should have a diet rich in the foods that supply the material needed for building muscle and hormones. We need protein to build muscle and fat for building hormones. A diet rich in healthy proteins and healthy fats is important. Foods such as nuts, beans, eggs, fish, some red meat, chicken, raw dairy products (limit amounts of processed dairy), and then add in oils such as coconut oil, butter, and olive oil. If you eat plenty of foods that already contain their own fat, you do not have to worry so much about adding in extra.

It takes approximately 12 months: to replace EVERYTHING, even our bones and teeth! Keep in mind, this our current cell generation gives birth to the new generation, so this does NOT mean the next generation with be without defects. For the health of our bones, joints and connective tissue, we need an active lifestyle; weight bearing exercises for the large muscle groups along with a diet rich in calcium, with the addition of vitamin D supplementation, (if you do not get adequate sun exposure), vitamin D helps our body absorb calcium.

Have you ever had muddy or rusty water come into your home's plumbing network? If you have, you probably remember that you had to give it a little time to let the good clean water clean and clear the bad water out of the plumbing system. Since our new generations of cells are a product of the parent generation of cells, we have to give it some time for healthy lifestyle choices to clear the effects of bad lifestyle habits. Healthy lifestyle choices help us clear muddy water!

Simple steps to building a new you: When we empower our body by cleansing it, then adding good lifestyle habits (while eliminating the bad), our body can become younger in the way it conducts itself as well as lower our need for man made chemicals and supplementation. This will help revitalize everything from our skin cells to the cells that make up our vital organs, turning our body and its systems into a defender against chronic disease and premature aging instead of a magnet for it!

Why look externally for the fountain of youth and healing, when it was designed within us? This fountain produces trillions of cells every year, and the health of these cells is largely determined by the daily lifestyle choices we make! Do you want to give this cellular fountain, muddy or clean water to produce your next generation of cells?

A lot of time is spent in pursuit of the fountain of youth that could be spent on empowering the healthy cellular fountain of youth within us!

Our body is made up of around 2 trillion cells; our body produces around 10 billion cells a day...

Million: 1,000,000

Billion: 1,000,000,000

Trillion: 1,000,000,000,000

A million seconds is 13 days

A billion seconds is 31 years

A trillion seconds is 31,688 years

Hormonal Disruption!

 This morning I was listening to the news and one of the first things that caught my attention was a recent study on "early menopause being triggered by some common household chemicals." These chemicals can affect our nervous system, our hormonal system, our immune system and our detoxification system as well.

 Could hormone imbalances possibly have far reaching effects in helping spawn some of the most pervasive chronic diseases? It appears so to me...

 Example: heart disease is the number one killer and even the heart is a part of the endocrine (hormone production) system. This was not known until the 1980's and lead to the groundbreaking discovery that the heart produces hormones into the blood that help the heart govern blood pressure and volume, wow can you imagine your body naturally doing something like that?

Hormones being disrupted by environmental exposures, skin products, hormones in our food and food additives would not be considered a new thing, but it is good to know that publicity is shedding some light on this issue. When we look at the abnormal fast development of children which has become the new normal and now the younger age in menopause, (it doesn't take a rocket scientist to figure out that something un-natural JUST MIGHT be developing from the massive increased usage of unnatural products!

The EPA has an Endocrine Disrupter Screening Program (EDSP) and in 2012 released a list of 10,000 chemicals, (this document is 176 pages of chemicals and there are actually around 85,000 chemicals on the market). How can they keep up with the effects of these chemicals, especially when used in combination with others?

This was in a New York Times article April 13, 2013: "In its history, the E.P.A. has mandated safety testing for only a small percentage of the 85,000 industrial chemicals available for use today. And once chemicals are in use, the burden on the E.P.A. is so high that it has succeeded in banning or restricting only five substances, and often only in specific applications: polychlorinated biphenyls, dioxin, hexavalent chromium, asbestos and chlorofluorocarbons."

Excuse a little personal rant, but isn't it weird how hard it is for an agency (that at its origin was set up to protect the people), has really stringent guidelines curbing them from banning toxic chemicals (to protect the public), but the USDA and the FDA along with our politicians have no problem in setting it up so that a food like milk cannot be bought, sold and consumed like it was for thousands of years? Or that an herbal plant (such as marijuana) that has many medicinal benefits gets scrutinized far more then drugs the FDA has put their stamp of approval on that has caused death and addiction on a mass scale? It probably isn't nearly so much to do with safety, as it is for industrial monopolization and for creating a taxable funnel for products that could otherwise be produced and traded among free people in a free market.

We can drive ourselves nuts, (trying to figure out what all the bad things around us are and what we need to stay away from), or we can simply limit our exposure. Its a lot like studying counterfeits, its simply much easier to learn the real thing then trying to learn every new counterfeit that hits the market. And when it comes to our food, household cleaners and skincare products, the same method applies.

Oft times hormone imbalances can be the cause of problem fatty areas as well and since fat helps absorb these toxins to protect the rest of the body, our fatty deposits can be a holding area for a lot of toxicity. That's a big reason, that weight loss should be incorporated with lots of water and a high fiber diet to pass these toxins out in our waste and to keep us from reabsorbing them.

A January 28-2015, Natural News article stated that, "It is estimated that there are over 80,000 toxic chemicals used regularly in the US. There are over 500 chemicals stored in our body and the average individual has at least seven pesticides tested in their urine."

Although it sounds bad when all these chemicals are found in the urine, it does show that the body is trying to get rid of foreign and hazardous material. If we can empower that system, (colon, liver, kidneys and skin) we can lead deflective lives and not worry so much about the things that swirl around us. To do this, we have to stay active, drink plenty of water, eat good fiber rich nutrition and keep our antioxidant levels high in the blood, (fruits, vegetables and nuts are a great source for that).

Keeping your house well ventilated when you're cleaning, (especially when using toxic chemicals) can help lower environmental toxins in your home. Toxic cleaners may make your house smell clean, but your body doesn't think it does!

Last but not least, stress is a bad hormone disrupter and is a big cause of belly fat. Mental stress causes an imbalance in cortisol when it's not countered with physical stress. Resistance training with weights and high intensity interval training to the point that you feel the burn really helps balance hormones.

 Keeping a good diet, plenty of water, and an active lifestyle will help us to eliminate and deflect the bad instead of being a toxin sponge!

This Little Pump Inside Our Chest

Our heart pumps around 20 quarts of blood per minute (at rest) and will pump a total of around 1.5 million gallons of blood (into a network of approximately 50,000 miles of blood vessels) every year for us! This little fist size pump is an amazing source of life for the rest of our body, and without its continued supply of oxygenated, nutrient carrying blood; our state of affairs will deteriorate fast!

February is American Heart Month and is used to increase our awareness of cardiovascular disease and what we can do to prevent not only death and slowed performance from heart related complications, but to help us increase cardiovascular performance!

Cardiovascular disease, (which includes heart disease, stroke, and high blood pressure) is the number 1 killer of women and men in the United

States, and the answer is not more medicine, the answer is in correcting what is aggravating our heart and cardiovascular system, such as diets loaded with sugar and high fructose corn syrup, lack of exercise, stress, and lack of deep sleep!

Our blood pump (heart) is nestled in the middle of our chest between two large oxygen pumps (our lungs) and keeping these three healthy is not only a life or death issue, it can mean the difference in everything from helping prevent chronic disease to things such as our energy levels. When our oxygen levels drop, so does our energy and our capability to fight chronic disease.

Example: cancer hates oxygen. Cancer is very anaerobic (likes to work with sugar, not oxygen and fat).

Since our heart works so silently, and steadily within us, we oft times take it for granted until we get some pretty severe warning signs that it is getting tired of our crappy treatment. Sometimes with proper care, we can turn things around, but if neglected for too long, it can cause death and at the least, decreased performance from the damage.

There are simply no substitutes for the basic healthy lifestyle habits that our heart wants, and until we start looking at our complications as a definition for the underlying problem and then correct this, the relationship between our heart and us is going to get worse.

Example: when we take a blood pressure medicine without trying to find out why our vascular system is under pressure, it's like putting a muzzle on our husband or wife when they're upset and then acting like they got no complaint!

The basic healthy habits still work for maintaining, and often times can even help in restoring health to your heart and cardiovascular system.

These basics are: fresh clean air, heart healthy balanced diet, sunshine, staying hydrated with clean water, exercise, deep rest, sleep, stress release, fun, and quality time spent with the ones you care about!

When we give back to this pump inside us that tirelessly continues to push oxygen, hydration and nutrients out to our body, it will oft times thank us in long term peak performance!

Why has Heart Disease Become The Number One Killer?

If we do not ask ourselves this simple question, (just like we should ask ourselves why has cancer become the number 2 leading killer), we will continue to treat a never ending supply of symptoms that will be continually generated from a common source. It's like spending time, money, resources, energy and tons of mental stress, mopping up water and refusing to go find the spigot that is generating the mess and simply turning it off. And in this case, THE PRIMARY SPIGOT FOR HEART DISEASE IS DIET & INACTIVITY!

This chapter is simply to bring awareness to a disease that has about a 100% chance of taking us out, or someone close to us.

According to the American Heart & Stroke Association's "Heart Disease and Stroke Statistics

Update," about 2,150 Americans die each day from cardiovascular death and it is the number one cause of death in the world.

In 2012 Dr. Dwight Lundell a heart surgeon that has performed over 5,000 open-heart surgeries stated that, "despite the fact that 25% of the population takes expensive statin medications and despite the fact we have reduced the fat content of our diets, more Americans will die of heart disease than ever before."

The American Heart Association and the American College of Cardiology's answer in 2014 was to make statins available to many millions more by making it easier to qualify for these drugs, (such as ones who don't yet have a cholesterol problem), but are in a group that is considered an increased risk. But then these are probably the same ones that advised a low fat diet with very little precautions on sugars, artificial sweeteners and grain products for the past 40 years.

We have trillions of cells that make up our body and according to the Mayo Clinic, cholesterol is found in every cell of the body, yet we are consuming massive amounts of cholesterol lowering drugs and crossing our fingers in hopes there will not be repercussions to other functions of the body as well as long term side effects. After all, shouldn't we be asking ourselves what is causing cholesterol to stick to our veins and arteries? Could it be because of injury???

A high sugar diet (which we now have loads of diabetic drugs to help compensate) will aggravate the lining of our blood vessel walls. Imagine taking some steel wool and scrubbing a spot on your body several times a day, every day. After a while it will turn red from inflammation and the ensuing healing process and if this happens for long enough and the injury goes deep enough, it is apt break through our skin and even if we stop, part of the healing process is the forming of a scab. But if we take care of this area, after a while, the scab will start flaking off (and disappearing) as the new healthy skin forms underneath. We encourage this healing process by being nice to the scabbing area, not by taking anti-scabbing medicine.

It simply makes sense to me that low-density cholesterol (LDL), is sticking to our arteries and veins because of injury (from our high sugar and artificial sweetener diets). Is it not logical to think that the hardening of our arteries and plaque is from continuous injury? And what we consider bad cholesterol (LDL) is our arteries and veins trying to protect themselves from what we're consuming? So shouldn't we look for what is causing the Low Density Lipids (LDL) to line our arteries and veins before we try to lower it with pills? Isn't that like striping our armor off during conflict?

The primary conflict our heart, arteries and veins face is a constant stream of sugars and processed foods in our diet, inactivity, too much stress, and not enough deep sleep.

Foods That Help Our Heart Tick

Keeping ourselves surrounded with heart healthy foods for our meals and snacks can be a great defense in not only warding off heart disease, but can help us create a highly energized environment for our heart and vascular system as well!

Cholesterol has been considered the bad guy for our heart and artery systems for years, but now we're discovering that our body just may be using it for healing and protecting veins and arteries that are hurting from a high sugar diet. Inflammation seems to be the reason now, but something is causing the inflammation. Cutting sugar (especially refined sugar and starches from processed food) can help us soothe the linings of our arteries and blood vessels, giving them a good reason to start dissolving this protective layer of cholesterol and plaque.

Cholesterol is used for trillions of cells in our body, so we also shouldn't be surprised that our body likes saturated fats to make this cholesterol from, after all it's the form of fat in real food, (eggs, meat, nuts, avocados, coconuts etc.).

There is a list of foods, spices etc. that have risen to the top that appear to have a positive impact on our heart and its systems.

As a disclaimer: this is simply the ones I would want to use for strengthening my heart, for better blood circulation and to protect myself from cardiovascular disease.

Pomegranate: for reduction of atherosclerosis/ plaque, and to stimulate production of nitric oxide, which helps with healthy blood flow).

Kale: for prevention of atherosclerosis/ plaque.

Avocado: for lowering LDL cholesterol and increase HDL cholesterol.

Whole grains, beans and other high fiber foods: for helping lower cholesterol through the removal of bile in digestion. When fiber drags bile out through our waste, our liver has to make new bile (we use it to digest fat) and it makes this new replacement bile from cholesterol.

Healthy fats: from olive oil, coconut oil, nuts, fish and unprocessed dairy, for building the cells of our blood and blood vessels.

Persimmons: for lowering LDL cholesterol and triglycerides.

Oranges: for reduction in blood pressure, cholesterol and antioxidants to improve blood vessel function and prevention of heart failure. I like oranges in their fruit form much more then the processed juice.

Cranberries: for reducing overall risk of heart disease.

Dark Colored Berries: for Resveratrol and its cardio friendly antioxidant effect.

Red wine or Dark beer: for the polyphenols to help keep blood vessels flexible and to reduce clotting.

Cheese, and butter: from grass fed dairy (for inhibiting atherosclerosis, reducing levels of circulating blood fats and to normalize impaired glucose uptake).

Watermelon, Spinach, Lentils, Dark Chocolate and Apple Cider Vinegar: for lowering blood pressure.

Fish rich in omega-3 fatty acids (for lowering triglycerides and increasing HDL)

Red vegetables and fruits: for lowering risk of stroke, prevention of blood clots and for improving blood circulation.

Cayenne Pepper: for rapidly equalizing blood pressure in the arterial and venous system - it warms the body - dilates blood vessels -increases circulation and blood flow to all major organs which facilitates oxygen and nutrient delivery.

Green Tea: for lowering cholesterol, maintaining healthy circulation, promotes healthy teeth and gums as well as for overall heart health).

Garlic: for inhibiting and decreasing atherosclerosis/ plaque in the arteries.

Cinnamon for helping reduce blood fats and plaque build up by helping control blood glucose levels. Also for its anti-inflammatory benefits that I feel would extend to the blood vessel walls.

Arginine: for dilating and relaxing blood, improved circulation through nitric oxide production.

Mediterranean Diet: the diet I would want to be on if I was diagnosed with heart disease.

Positive emotions, exercise and staying stress free are also great medicine for the heart!

I hope you live a heart friendly lifestyle, not only to prevent heart disease, but also to live your life with strength, vitality and endurance!

Renewing Our Worn Out Joints

Life brings a certain amount of wear and tear to our body, but due to our body's amazing capability to repair itself, oft times all we feel is a little temporary pain or weakness and then it goes away (and usually toughens up slightly). Most times all we have to do is favor this particular body part and give it some extra rest and it will heal on its own.

The CDC says that 1 in 2 people may develop symptomatic osteoarthritis by age 85. It also says that two in three people who are obese may develop symptomatic knee osteoarthritis in their lifetime. We probably should connect the dots on this one!

Wear and tear without recovery time does not yield good results. Our body adapts to stress, but it needs recovery time to fix day-to-day stress (especially stresses it is not accustomed to) and sometimes we need extra recovery time when we really gave our joints, tendons and ligaments the shaft!

Acute inflammation: sometimes life gets in the way of proper recovery time and if we're not careful this can lead to inflammation in the area that is getting aggravated repeatedly. This inflammation is a part of the healing process, but it gives out a pain signal due to the puffy tissue it has created around the affected area (to speed the recovery process). Pain is a good thing, because it tells us to let up, pull back, lighten up, limp, brace ourselves etc.

Chronic inflammation: when an area continues to get aggravated, this acute inflammation can turn into chronic inflammation and yield a diseased area. This can lead to arthritic conditions of our joints, in much the same way that it will produce cancer, heart, brain and many other chronic diseases.

There are a few things we can do to help lighten the load around our joints and even help build back our joint health even if we are told we have to have surgery;

Weight loss: this can ease the burden on our joints, especially for a person that doesn't have strong muscles supporting their weight. Losing extra pounds helps lift a performance burden off of our skeletal system as well as our supporting organ system.

Exercise: when we strengthen muscles around our joints as well as our core, it helps split the workload on the joint area. When muscle isn't toned and strengthened, we become like dead weight to our bones, joints, tendons and ligaments. Consistent exercise, with good range of motion also stimulates the production of synovial fluid in our joint areas, (this is our joint grease).

Have you ever been helping someone lift something, only to look over and realize the person that is supposed to be splitting the load with you is barely helping? In life that is aggravating and it's no different for what our joints expect from the surrounding muscles.

Someone that is a very active heavy person can have good joint health due to the body's capability for adaption. The problem is when a person is inactive or becomes inactive and their muscles shrink down and become weak and are not doing their fair share of the work.

Recovery: resting weary overworked joints is one of the greatest remedies for what ails our joints tendons and ligaments.

Foods and nutrients good for bone and joint health:

Apples, grapes, almonds, peanuts and coconut oil: for bone health and guarding against osteoarthritis.

Omega-3 rich fish such as Norwegian sardines, Atlantic mackerel, rainbow trout, or striped bass: for controlling systemic inflammation.

Sesame seeds, and cayenne pepper: for arthritic pain. Sesame seeds have been shown to be as effective as Tylenol for arthritic pain.

Good quality protein and fat sources: for building muscle to support our skeletal structure.

Good add-ins: calcium, vitamin D, vitamin C, turmeric, glucosamine and chondroitin, and bone broth (this one has a lot of other health benefits as well). Of course one of my favorites for bone health and protein support is raw dairy milk, (however corporate and political cronyism has made this one illegal in most states).

Using joint supports: if you have joint problems, (low back, knee, elbow etc.) wear a support for that area and try to do things to make it feel better by figuring out what it wants instead of trying to do things that help us not feel its pain. If we figure out what will help our hurting joint wants instead of taking anti-inflammatory medicine, pain blocks and medications, (that simply tell these areas that are hurting, to shut up), our body parts will oft times thank us by actually healing.

Example: if you are in touch with the pain in your hip, you will probably limp, but if you take pain medicine and walk like regular, (since you cannot feel the pain the hip is in), it will probably be hurting worse the next day.

Why is it that people who are told, they HAVE TO HAVE back or knee surgery, are immediately upon diagnosis prescribed pain pills, pain blocks, and anti-inflammation drugs instead of a back belt, decompression therapy, knee support, and joint building supplements (between diagnosis and time of surgery)? But then why would a salesman want to show you how you can avoid doing business with him?

Hormonal Fatty Deposits

Did you know that hormones can help the body decide where it should store fat? It does, and it starts for most of us during our young years, especially around puberty.

Prior to this, male and female shape is much the same. Body fat is primarily what makes the difference in shape between males and females.

Hormones are like traffic cops in our body, that tell organs and cells how to react to certain things.

Example: when we get an increase of sugar in our blood, our pancreas will release insulin to safely remove the excess sugars and carry it off to various places of the body to store it. I often tell my members, that if we have extra stored body fat, its only because the insulin is doing its job, (sugar left in the blood can cause our arteries and blood vessels become a sticky mess).

Hormones that can affect fatty deposits: estrogen, cortisol, low testosterone, high testosterone, high insulin, low progesterone, low growth hormone, low DHEA.

Keeping our hormones in balance can go a long ways in helping keep body fat levels down and to help distribute it throughout our body, in a way that we want. Body fat under the skin can help us look better and is not a bad thing at all. It's when we get too much that it begins to present a problem.

All these hormones and what they do, can really be complicated to remember, and I am not advocating at all that someone needs to learn them. You can get blood work done to see if you have hormone imbalances, but there are some simple things we should do before we feel we should spend the time and money getting blood work done. Remember, there is a reason hormones get out of whack and we should figure out what that is before we force hormonal changes synthetically!

These are great hormone balancers:

1. Water as beverage of choice

2. Healthy diet with unprocessed foods

3. Weight control

4. Exercise and activity

5. Sunshine

6. Clean unpolluted air

7. Healthy social connections

8. Deep sleep

9. Staying mentally stress free or finding ways to get rid of it.

Hormonal fatty deposits for women:

Chest fat: high estrogen, low testosterone.

Belly fat: high cortisol, high insulin, low or high estrogen, high testosterone, low growth hormone.

Love handle fat: high insulin and blood sugar imbalance.

Hips, butt and thigh fat: high estrogen, low progesterone, low growth hormone.

Hormonal fatty deposits for men:

Chest fat: high estrogen, low testosterone.

Arm fat: high insulin, low DHEA.

Abdominal fat: high insulin, high estrogen, high cortisol, and low growth hormone.

Love handle fat: high insulin, blood sugar imbalance.

Hips, butt and thigh fat: high estrogen, low growth hormone.

Steps to track hormone imbalance:

1. Find out the possible hormonal imbalance for that area.

2. Find out what the hormones are for.

3. Find out what helps offset this hormone imbalance.

These 3 steps should help you track down where the problem may be coming from and what you can do to counter balance it.

Example for testosterone, growth hormone, cortisol and insulin:

Growth hormone: a higher rep set (where you go slow on the negative part of the rep), to make your muscles really feel the lactic acid burn, will increase growth hormone.

Testosterone: a heavier weight where your muscle fatigues (before you feel the lactic acid burn) boosts testosterone levels.

Cortisol: regular exercise and good sleep habits can help keep stress levels down, thus reducing cortisol levels.

Insulin: lowering our sugar intake, regular exercise (along with the extra muscle mass that comes with exercise), will help lower blood glucose levels, thus lowering insulin levels.

Insulin and cortisol: insulin spikes from sugar, and cortisol spikes from stress are 2 major culprits in causing fat deposits. Avoiding sweet foods and stress help shrink fatty deposits. If you cannot avoid stress, the endorphins from exercise will help offset the stress hormone cortisol and adrenaline hormones.

We could get lost in the maze of technical terms of hormones and body chemistry, but most hormonal issues can be remedied by

1. What we eat.

2. Exercise.

3. Sleep habits.

4. Keeping our stress levels down.

When we do these things with consistency, things start balancing out and fatty deposits start disappearing.

Our hormone systems have a feedback loop, (that can carry back a healthy message or a continued negative message), and the message for more or less production of the hormones they produce largely depends on us and our lifestyle choices...

What Soil Is Your Health and Fitness Planted In?

If our health and fitness were a seed, what kind of soil are we asking it to grow in? If we keep it surrounded by fast food, sugar, cigarette smoke, and a constant stream of pharmaceutical drugs, can we really expect it to produce good fruit? Is this not like expecting a recipe for a chocolate cake to produce a vanilla one?

Becoming a product of our surroundings is pretty exciting if we think about how rapidly our body builds another generation of cells to replace the trillions of cells that make up our body, or in how our muscles adapt to the stress we put our muscles under during exercise by making them larger, stronger and with more tone, definition and capability.

Garden of disease: if we could have a time lapse video of a person that gets off work from a job he or she has a bad attitude toward, (and who goes home each day after work and drinks alcohol until bedtime with a fast food supper, topped off with a muscle relaxer and sleep medicine), it's not hard to imagine what this person may look and feel like in 6 months.

Garden of health and fitness: if this same person starts waking up earlier, eats a healthy breakfast, packs a healthy lunch, starts treating their job and people he or she works with, with appreciation, gets off work and hits the gym, it's not hard to imagine the huge difference that could be made in even a 3 month period! After 6 months even more benefits start appearing and after a year the changes would be so stark that it almost would look like someone turned back the aging clock on the person. It's no different for an individual then it is for a plant that is put in fertile, moisturized dirt vs. hard, nutrient deficient, dry dirt.

Imagine how a tree would feel if it were not getting much water and the nutrient level was very low in the surrounding dirt, and we would trim the pale, blighted leaves and branches off to make it a healthier tree. That's how our body feels if we cut, medicate and radiate without changing what is actually causing the problem. It's like smashing the check engine light on our car and then acting like the problem is gone.

Example: taking a pain pill for a hurting hip (instead of using a crutch) and then walking around like this body part isn't hurting. This body part wants you to limp, and take the pressure of its regular load off of it for a while and let the inflammation and our other healing mechanisms do its duties. It does NOT want us to take anti-inflammatory medicine to mess up the healing process and pain pills to disconnect us from what it is going through. If you have to take a pain pill, at the least continue to lighten the load on the hip.

 Each choice we make, (whether its clogging up the oxygen we breath, with cigarette smoke vs. clean air, bad diet vs. healthy diet, active lifestyle vs. sedentary lifestyle, sunshine vs. chemical sun blockers, soda's and other high sugar, fructose, aspartame drink products vs. water, and social isolation vs. social connection) determines the soil our health is rooted in.

Our health and fitness has roots, and it is planted squarely in the lifestyle habits we choose and oft times the environment we select. This defines the outcome much like nutrient rich soil and hydration does for a plant. Each choice we make determines the dirt our health and fitness is planted in.

Restoring Old Fat aka Cellulite

Have you ever wondered why the fat under the skin on a younger person oft times looks much better then the fat under an older person's skin? One thing we know for sure is we appreciate dimples in our upper set of cheeks much more then we do the lower one! We know the culprit is cellulite, but what causes cellulite?

Cellulite is to fat like the wrinkle is to skin. If we take care of our skin, the elasticity will be better for much longer and if we keep our subcutaneous (under the skin) fat healthy, it will stay much smoother and help us avoid what we know as cellulite.

Men get cellulite too, however the reason cellulite is not as obvious in men, is most men have thicker skin, the fat is stored a little deeper, and fatty deposit areas differ from men and women (this is what makes our shapes different from each other).

Men are more apt to see cellulite form around the neck or abdominal areas.

The thing that is frustrating about cellulite, is many times during weight loss, it becomes even more obvious, due to loss of healthier surrounding fat that may have been covering it up. This is because our body is going to pull from the most accessible energy source and if it doesn't have a good blood supply our body's capability of fat transport from that area is not as good. Once we know what can make the older fat more accessible for our body to break it down for energy, we should then know what to do to get rid of our cellulite. Cellulite is like broken fat, so I like to think of this as fat repair...

Repairing broken fat: cellulite is blood and oxygen starved fat. Oxygen is the most vital nutrient to life and we know that blood is the transport system that delivers oxygen and the other nutrients that keep our body parts and its systems healthy!

Building a better blood flow: it is reasonable to assume, (if we get a better blood supply to our fatty deposits) that we should be able to burn fat from these areas better. Fat cells are like cans of food in that they both hold calories. Increasing blood flow would be like clearing a path in our storage pantry so we can get to some food that has been stored for a while and hasn't been in rotation like the cans of food in the front. Cellulite is like the dusty cans of food stuck behind the new and fresh cans of food.

Building muscle: this is a great way to increase blood flow to an area, so strength training and building muscle in the cellulite problem areas should help with the blood flow and the subsequent oxygenation of these areas. Building muscle keeps body parts from looking flabby as well; fat simply does not look so bad if there is toned muscle underneath. When we go on a crash diet, the loss of muscle can cause areas of our body to lose underlying firmness, oft times the upper layer of subcutaneous fat and skin simply mirrors what is happening underneath. Building muscle, through strength training and a good diet will help firm these areas.

Heat: heat will encourage blood flow into an area. Applying heat to a problem area of cellulite should encourage blood flow and increase our capability to use it as a source of energy.

Skin brushing: this is a good way to encourage blood flow into an area and is one that I certainly advocate. Simply get a brush that has plastic balls at the end (so it will not scratch or scuff your skin) and work this area in a circular motion periodically. You do not want to overdo this as this can make your skin hurt if you do too much at one time.

A combination of the 3 above methods will work great along with an antioxidant rich diet of fruits and vegetables and plenty of water!

This article was not to help figure out a new way to burn fat, but rather to promote either the healthy upkeep of the fat or restoring health to our fat cells. Remember, healthy fat under our skin helps keep our skin looking healthy, smooth, and young, after all, isn't our subcutaneous fat a big part of what our skin is planted on?

Bottom to the Top!

Most that know me, know that I get perturbed by things around us that need to be changed, whether it's BIG Pharma trying to become kingpins in chronic disease management, modern diet and food logistics, and of course a political system with a huge shortage of real statesmen and women, that simply add fuel to all the above. I'm beginning to see that our biggest hope for change at the top, is change at the bottom that forces change all the way through a system that has been corrupted by financial gain.

I was reminded of this fiasco recently, when watching the news on how painfully some of our state representatives came to the table and voted in favor of an extract from a God given herbal plant that could help with all kinds of conditions that modern medicine has been treating and most certainly would have liked to continue to have exclusivity for. Who would have thought that something herbal may work better then an entire series of laboratory produced knockoffs?

Unfortunately this plant is used by some for the sole purpose of getting high, just as alcohol is used by many to get drunk, however one has lots of medicinal use, the other has virtually none.

A while back I was watching a documentary on food and food logistics, and they brought out a point that really made sense, "we the consumer (there are several 100 million of us) hold the purse strings and what we choose to buy can have a big impact on market demands. And instead of worrying about creating change at the top, we should simply create change around ourselves, in what we purchase to eat." There is change happening and you can see it, by the new farmers markets that are springing up to meet the demands of consumers trying to eat healthier.

Have you noticed how (throughout the past 20-50 years); the 1000's of NEW FOODS have caused the middle section of grocery stores to swell up? Have you noticed over the past 5 years how that many of the nicer grocery stores are putting more emphasis into freshening up the look of the outer ring (fruits, vegetables, nuts, berries, meats, eggs and dairy sections) of the store? This keeps people coming into their stores for produce instead of the local produce stand or farmers market.

We can increase the availability of these foods, by purchasing from our neighbor's garden, the local roadside produce stands and our area farmer's market. We can put pressure on our representatives that stand guard over laws that represent crony capitalism, such as ones that prohibit the purchase and the sale of a food that is 1000's of years old, (raw milk).

February 19, 2014 the FDA submitted a letter to the Agricultural Committee of Georgia on the dangers of raw to help them defuse an attempt by people in Georgia for the right to buy and sell raw milk. The report could make someone (that was not connected to the dairy or nutrition industry) think raw milk was very hazardous to one's health. This really shows the desperation of the jugglers of information in an attempt to get our representatives to lazily accept what they say, instead of figuring out what they base their research on and see how it compares to other things the FDA readily allows and condones use of that has caused lots of death and destruction of health. The FDA testimony letter did not bother to say that the food in question (milk) has been consumed for 1000's of years in its raw state and only in the past 50 years, started causing problems such as lactose intolerance etc. Could it be that pasteurized for your safety, is not as healthy as it is in its raw, natural state? If it's so safe, why was death caused by consumption of Blue Bell ice cream recently? When was the last time you heard of a death caused by raw milk?

This particular law is the worst one I know, but its only one of many (connected to a powerful money and lobbyist trail) and is simply indicative of what happens when governmental agencies turn on the people they are supposed to serve and protect, by using laws created by our politicians that were designed to serve and protect corporate interests. Why would a dairyman fear a phone call from someone he or she does not know that wants to purchase raw milk from his dairy? If you cannot freely purchase or sell a food product that people have used in its raw state for 1000's of years, that's not freedom, that's tyranny! What you choose to put between your two lips should be your choice, we certainly have the right to smoke cigarettes, consume alcohol, carbonated-caffeinated-sugar and aspartame loaded sodas, but then they are controlled, packaged and taxable, right? It's an established fact that smoking cigarettes is one of the leading causes of death, yet it's legal, right?

I think its pretty clear to most of us by now, that change is not going to happen at the top unless the soil (that gives problems a root system to grow in) changes! Your purchases, your vote, your lifestyle is this soil and what grows on top represents you! Even though our action or inaction may seem like a little pebble dropped in a massive lake, the ripple effect can last a lifetime and longer! Sometimes change has to happen at the bottom, for change to happen at the top...

Functional Training for Real Life Function

Functional training is one of my favorite subjects, and is definitely my favorite way of teaching exercise programs. Functional training is simply empowering your every day movements, whether you're an athlete trying to strengthen his or her game or a senior strengthening mobility, stability and flexibility.

Training in this manner is not for increasing the size and power in one particular muscle group, but rather multiple muscle groups strengthened and trained together. This creates flow from one muscle group to the next vs. stiff blocky movement that happens with muscles that are trained separately instead of together.

Example: a bodybuilder that is trying to increase size of shoulders may set in a shoulder press unit that will protect his or her back while pressing dumbbells repeatedly overhead, however, someone that is trying to increase functional strength, will do exercises such as reaching down to the floor and picking up a barbell or a set of dumbbells and pushing it/them overhead.

 In real life, we don't have a seat or machine protecting our back when we lift, pull or press things, so why would an athlete or someone trying to enhance capabilities in real life train any different then how they move in real life, whether it's performance on track and field or simply doing yard work?

 Going into a gym, purchasing exercise equipment or simply using bodyweight exercises can be a little intimidating when someone is trying to figure it all out, but not so, if you are simply trying to improve real life function. By mimicking real life movements and using exercises to create a greater resistance (such as using a barbell or set of dumbbells while doing a squat) we simply build more powerful movements and greater endurance!

Example: If you always carry a heavy set of dumbbells (or other form of resistance) up and down a hill or stairs, eventually going up and down this hill or stairs with only your bodyweight will be super easy!

 Example bodyweight exercise: get down on the floor (use a chair or sofa if needed) and lay flat on the floor with arms stretched out overhead, then stand back up and extend arms overhead once again. Repeat until it becomes a slight strain to stand back up. Over a period of several weeks, you will see this become easy and your muscles used for this will become more toned and conditioned. You can use cans of food or dumbbells to increase resistance.

 Example barbell exercise: lift a barbell with weights up from the floor to your chest, then go into a full squat and as you stand back up, press the weight overhead.

 Training in this way teaches our muscles to work together. Bodybuilders pump individual muscle groups to increase size and strength; athletes train multiple groups of muscles at one time, to work together for more powerful and coordinated movements.

Never let a gym or exercise routine intimidate you into thinking you have to figure it out, simply use the contraptions it provides to serve the purpose you need it for. When you take real life movements and add resistance and duration to the movement in your exercise routine, it makes the movements and duties in real life become lighter and easier!

April (Cancer Control Month)?

When did the language start to change, from "The search for a cure" to "Cancer Control?"

 Controlling cancer is a great thing and is something we should be empowering our body to do the other 335 days of the year as well. But what are the ones behind a month dedicated to it advocating? A good way to figure this out is if the advocacy group or organization is putting healthy lifestyle habits first or if it's early detection. It's simple as that. If you are feeling a greater pull toward early detection then you are in prevention through healthy habits, then you have fallen prey to an industry that has a BIG need to keep you in its cycle of expensive drugs, office visits and diagnostic machines that they have spent a fortune on developing or purchasing.

 Is there a better way to build an industry off of chronic disease then to use fear mongering and being at the root of every conceivable awareness month possible? If we were screened for everything there was an awareness month for we would probably be radiated and eventually screened and stressed to death!

This morning when I was looking at a cancer calendar, I counted 29 different cancers and their respective Awareness Month or Awareness Week. This is enough to make someone feel like they're walking through a poison maze, never knowing which one they are going to become a victim too, much less knowing what is the best course of action to take for treatment. Most of these individual cancers have their own fields of research, screenings and medicine to help manage the disease. So when you get into all the research, all the diagnostics, and the latest greatest pharmaceutical cancer treatments and try to figure out what your best course of action is, it can be mind-boggling. It makes me really thankful for the simple healthy fundamentals that don't change, and still will prevent, shrink and even eliminate the bad stuff!

Making it simple: almost all-chronic disease, (including most cancers) has a common denominator... LIFESTYLE HABITS!!!

1. Bad lifestyle habits are cancerous.

2. Good lifestyle habits help the body do what it does best, and that is to heal itself and prevent cancer!

It's much easier learning and keeping good lifestyle habits, then spending a lifetime in the search for an elusive cure. Should we really expect the same groups (that stay in existence because of a disease) to produce a cure and put themselves and their affiliates out of business?

Our body is a cell factory: we are made up of trillions of cells that are constantly getting replaced, and our body depends on us for the material it makes these cells out of. Our lungs, liver, colon, skin, brain and other systems of our body constantly produce cells to generate themselves. If one of these organs gets damaged, (from unhealthy diet, cigarette smoke etc.) but continues to produce cells, these damaged cells sometimes do not behave (and turn off growth) like the normal ones. The mess may build up and accumulate in that organ until it affects that organ's function. It may also leave that organ (metastasize) and become a part of another organ system that it has no business in and start affecting the way that assembly line (organ system) works. Imagine a deformed liver cell attaching itself to a spot in the kidney, how messed up is that?

Cancer Control: though lifestyle is linked to most cancers, we can take it a step further, as to what happens as a result of unhealthy lifestyle choices. Bad lifestyle choices simply cause oxidative stress to our cells much like the rusting that happens after a car is scratched past its protective paint layer (this scratch oxidizes and produces rust). This oxidation causes damage to our cells and is at the root of chronic diseases, including most cancer. Antioxidants help rid the body of this excess oxidation. This is why a diet rich in antioxidants (fruits, vegetables, nuts and berries) is one of the best ways to prevent and get rid of cancer. Balanced healthy diet, clean air, water, exercise, deep sleep, sunshine, and positive mindset is how we not only maintain our factory, but how we help repair and correct damage, so our body doesn't continue to produce abnormal cells.

The next few chapters will be on controlling cancer, and how your body can discover, target and prevent cancer on its own, after all your body is fighting cancer right now and will continue doing so, long before a man made diagnostic machine will discover and diagnose you to have cancer.

What are you doing or not doing to help your body win its fight against cancer?

Homeostasis vs. Cancer

Homeostasis is simply a state of normal that our body tries to return to no matter if we get dehydrated, cold, hot, sick, infections or even get emotionally upset. This list of things the body is continually trying to keep balanced is a long one and like many say... the struggle is real!

Our body is constantly trying to adjust to our environment, some of which are out of our control, but there is plenty we can do and by doing these, we help our body offset the bad things in our environment that we cannot control. We can help our body by doing things that synchronize it with the healthy things in our region, such as local grown foods vs. ones grown 1000's of miles away. If a food thrives in an area, it's quite obvious that this plant or this animal has homeostasis with this region. I am completely convinced that God designed nature this way, so it makes no sense to me to live off of food that does not live in the same environment that I do.

When we give our body healthy things to work with, it makes things much easier to keep in balance or bring back in balance. Giving our body unhealthy or foreign things to work with and expecting a good result is like giving a chef mangos and expecting him or her to be able to make a peach pie out of it!

The system of checks and balances is oft times quietly at work within us trying to normalize everything from the amount of acid in our stomach, to how things get interpreted by the brain after entering the eyeball(s). We can see the above two, by how our digestive tract reacts to bad or hard to digest food or how we sometimes have very different reaction when we see something compared to other times.

Cancer: our body is constantly fighting cancer by keeping things such as our pH (acid/alkaline) levels in balance. There seems to be some controversy in what effects this, but either way, just like chronic (continued) inflammation we should look at our body's over production of acid as a reaction to things it doesn't like and if we continue to do things to our body that causes it to produce acid, and inflammation, it can yield bad results. When there is continuous festering of our body's defense mechanisms, it can damage our DNA and cause it to give out warped blueprints to build new cells and these cells oft times grow in an unusual manner and sometimes do not stop when they're supposed to, thus yielding a growth we call cancer.

Immune system: whether our cancer is isolated or systemic, just like the feedback loops of a well armed security system, our immune system reads trouble spots and sends its specialists to that area to get rid of the problem.

Homeostasis: our body naturally sounds the alarm when things get out of whack and it will go to work to bring it back into normal balance. And whether cancer stays isolated in an area or metastasizes into other areas of the body, it is not considered normal, so if we have a strong immune system, it will increase the chances that it can discover the cancer on its own, long before its medically diagnosable state, and will shrink or eliminate it thus restoring health (homeostasis) in this tissue or organ area oft times without us even realizing the little hiccup on our immune system's radar screen.

Cancer is something that is hurting and stealing nutrients from a body part or body system and our immune system is not designed to hurt it further, but rather to get rid of what is causing the pain to this area and to stimulate the healing process and bring this area(s) back in synch with the rest of the body.

I apologize if it seems I repeat myself on the following (I admit it's intentional), but unlike many diagnostics and treatment protocols, (these don't change). These are the 6 healthy basics that still help (after 1000's of years with no bad side effects) to induce a homeostatic environment within us that is very unfriendly to cancer and other chronic disease...

1. Plenty of clean oxygen with deep breathing through exercise, cancer hates oxygen.

2. Plenty of oxygen loaded water; a well-hydrated and oxygenated body creates an unfriendly cancer environment.

3. Healthy diet with plenty of antioxidant rich fruits, vegetables, nuts, beans and berries, antioxidants help fight oxidation which is a primary source of cancer.

4. Regular exercise, this helps strengthen us and helps circulate and deliver items 1 - 3 above!

5. Sunshine in moderate doses and yes, sunshine is very healthy but just like exercise is healthy, 3 hours of exercise can be very unhealthy to our muscles, joints, tendons, ligaments, and kidneys-just as 3 hours of sunshine is very inflammatory to skin that isn't accustomed to even 30 minutes of sunshine! The sun is our primary source for the body's own production of vitamin D (a powerful cancer fighting hormone)!

6. Last but not least, deep sleep, relaxation and stress relief! This is when the body repairs damage.

Our body has powerful diagnostic tools and when they detect an imbalance, they have an exact designer prescription list to send to our immune system for nutrients, chemical reactions, and body generated drugs (and yes our body makes its own drugs) to help our body pull itself back into balance.

Question: what am I doing that is assisting or undermining the balance that my body is trying to maintain or return to?

Diagnosed To Death

In July of 2013 the Journal of the American Medical Association (JAMA) published an article from researchers at the National Institute of Cancer that caused quite a stir, "Over diagnosis and Over treatment in Cancer: An Opportunity for Improvement."

Excerpt: "In the case of an indolent [slow growing] tumor, detection is potentially harmful because it can result in over treatment... Physicians, patients, and the general public must recognize that over diagnosis is common and occurs more frequently with cancer screening. Over diagnosis, or identification of indolent cancer, is common in breast, lung, prostate, and thyroid cancer." **Esserman MD, et.al. JAMA 2013.108415**

One of the points this article brought out was that treatment of non-lethal disease increases the percentage of survival statistics. So what this is really saying is that cancer treatment protocols have been taking credit for survival rates from cases where the person would've survived on their own.

This is the last article in this cancer series and I do not want to spend your time on learning about a lucrative industry (that thrives off of fear for its continued treatment and diagnostic cycles), but rather on ways we can empower our own early detection system to prevent and eliminate cancer on its own. The causes of cancer are toxins and a weakened immune system, so if we can figure out what we do to help our body to naturally get rid of toxins and what can build up our immune system (instead of immune altering treatments such as chemotherapy), it just may help us give our body what it needs to prevent and even cure cancer instead of the seemingly illusive search for the cure.

These are the protocols I like, and I like to call them Nature's Oncology Prescription.

1. Oxygen. **2.** Detoxify. **3.** Organic diet. **4.** Rebounding.

1. Oxygen: getting as much oxygen into the cells of your body will help with detoxification and cancer absolutely hates oxygen! So whether through deep controlled breathing or through intense exercise that makes us huff and puff, it is very important to get lots of clean oxygen into our body and get the stale air and carbon dioxide out. Also exercising all areas of the body helps us to stimulate oxygen and nutrient rich blood flow to those areas.

2. Detox: when we detox it helps reset our system by getting rid of the sludge build up in our digestive tract, kidneys and liver. After we do this, our energy to do battle against chronic disease is much higher. When we hit the reset button on our detox organs (liver, kidneys and colon), they're much more capable to detoxify the rest of our body from years of toxic buildup. A good detox product that detoxifies liver, kidneys and colon can be helpful with this process. My favorite is the Lee

Haney 7 Day Systemic Cleansing Detox. Once this is over, our body's natural detox pathways can get rid of toxins as we shed them from the rest of the body (through dietary and other lifestyle changes). During any detox, it is important to have a high fiber diet, for proper elimination of these toxins, otherwise they'll absorb back into our system.

3. Organic diet: this may be aggravating to do, but if you're fighting cancer, you want to take in foods without the accompanying toxins and cancer causing carcinogens. The best way to do this is to know where your food comes from or grow it yourself. Keeping a diet with plenty of antioxidant rich fruits, vegetables, nuts, beans and berries; helps us lower oxidative stress and inflammation, which is a primary source of festering that leads to cancer. A diet with lots of organic fiber rich fruits and vegetables with plenty of clean water also helps as a continual detox.

4. Rebounding: our lymph system is our body's drainage system and it flows north not south. It brings our excess fluid back into circulation. But before doing this, it filters this fluid through the lymph nodes to kill any foreign invaders, (this is the reason our white blood cell count goes up when our body is fighting an infection or something). This specialized drainage system will form antibodies specifically designed to kill foreign invaders. Our lymph fluid moves upward through the lymph nodes and what stimulates this huge part of our immune system is up and down motion. So you can imagine how little our fluid moves through our lymph system when we set idle for long periods. We have about 2 times the amount of lymph fluid (in our lymphatic system) as we do blood, but it doesn't have a pump like our blood does, it relies on physical movement of our muscles. What really stimulates the movement of lymph fluids is up and down movement so one of the best stimulators for this huge part of our immune system is a small rebounder trampoline.

The avoid list:

1. Sugar.

2. Processed foods and drinks.

3. Poorly ventilated, low oxygen areas, extended times of sitting idle, inhaling fumes from household and other chemicals, cigarettes, alcohol, narcotics and other pharmaceutical drugs that could be eliminated through lifestyle change.

The 7 Best Doctors of Oncology are free:

1. Clean Oxygen.

2. Clean Water.

3. Healthy Diet.

4. Activity/Exercise.

5. Sunshine.

6. Sleep.

7. Positive Mindset!

I hope you stay not only physically free from cancer, but mentally free of the fear of cancer!

Burning Fat by Controlling Blood Sugar

Lowering blood sugar is one of the simplest strategies to trigger the fat burning process. Lowering our blood sugar simply helps our body recognize the need for another source of fuel, thus triggering the release of energy substance from our fat cells.

Having a high blood glucose level is very dangerous (because of things getting sticky), so our body has a series of triggers that it operates on to moderate the level of glucose in our blood.

When we take in high levels of sugar and starches (especially when we're not very active) our body often has no choice other then to store the extra sugars (in the form of fat) throughout our body, including our liver. This is set up this way so our body can feed itself when we cannot access food. However, when we constantly take in excess calories over the amount we burn off, it starts distorting our shape.

I really wish everyone that is trying to lose weight, would get a blood glucose monitoring kit to check blood sugar levels periodically. You can get them for around ($40) or for approximately the price of a bottle of fat burners. Checking your blood glucose levels regularly makes you want to eat slower digesting foods and strengthens your resolve against dumping sugar loads into your body!

Lowering blood sugar through diet: many of the foods we eat are converted to glucose so that we have fuel to burn for our energy needs, (the other nutrients are for keeping our blood strong, fighting disease and rebuilding our body). The secret lies in foods that break down slower.

Example: milkshake vs. sweet potato or an apple with a serving of nuts vs. a fruit smoothie. If you drink a liquid meal or shake, consume it over a longer period of time, so it won't all hit your system at one time, (this causes blood glucose spikes).

Our choice of foods goes a long way in keeping our blood sugar levels steady. It's the spikes in sugar that cause weight gain. Food fats are not the problem; sugar spikes from sugar-loaded foods, drinks and high starch meals are the primary cause of fatty deposits. This includes the entire family of sweeteners whether naturally occurring or chemically altered sugars. This includes fruits, constantly eating them, can keep blood glucose levels spiked, so that our body has difficulty switching to fat burn mode. Vegetable and nut snacks are much better for burning fat.

Sugar spikes insulin levels: when we have spiked insulin levels from a high sugar intake, it shuts off the fat burning process in our body. Sugar becomes the most necessary fuel to burn, (because having high levels of it in our blood can wreak havoc). After the large amount of insulin has transported our sugar off to various parts of our body, it will trigger the release of fat once again as an energy source, (the problem is, many of us take in just enough sugar to keep this fat burn process turned off, or at the least, not operating efficiently.

Dietary tip for burning body fat: if you want to learn what foods will help avoid sugar spikes, avoid fatty deposits, and help you burn body fat, get a list of foods that a type 2 diabetic can have. And do NOT drink sugar beverages with meals!

Lowering blood sugar through exercise: intense activity burns off our excess blood glucose. When we get the level low enough during exercise, it triggers the release of body fat and we start burning fat for energy. A secondary effect that regular exercise has (on blood sugar levels) is, the added muscle gives us better capability to suck up excess sugar from our blood and burn it off with all the activity that is happening inside all these muscle cells.

Avoiding sugar spikes not only helps us to burn fat, it also helps us prevent diabetes as well as control diabetes without insulin medications. Insulin usage without lifestyle change = obesity.

 If we all would eat like a type 2 diabetic would have to, (if he or she couldn't get medical insulin) we would be a much leaner society...

Burning Fat with
Apple Cider Vinegar

This is a slight continuation of that of the prior chapter "Burning Fat by Controlling Sugar Spikes" for the part apple cider vinegar seems to play in helping control blood sugar spikes.

I've personally been mixing apple cider vinegar in water and drinking it on an empty stomach (first thing in the morning), for quite some time now, because of all the health benefits that it is claimed to have. There has however been some research that has caught my attention for its benefits in potentially effecting weight loss, and the underlying reason is steady or lower blood glucose levels. When sugar gets spiked in the blood there are 3 things that can happen to the extra sugar:

1. We burn it off by exercising or other active physical movement.

2. Our blood carries it to the liver and converts it to triglycerides.

3. If it stays in the blood it can cause a sticky mess (aka diabetic complications)!

The continual spikes in sugar is what in turn spikes our insulin levels, turns off our fat burning switch, creates insulin resistance, and wears out our pancreas. So if there were something you could take prior to eating that might help (keep blood sugar levels steady, increase insulin sensitivity and take some burden off your pancreas), would it be worth a try?

The Journal of Functional Foods (2013) research showed that, consuming 1 tablespoon of apple cider vinegar in 8 oz. of water prior to mealtime, reduced fasting blood glucose concentrations in healthy adults at risk for type 2 diabetes.

Japanese study published in 2009 associated vinegar consumption with lower bodyweight, BMI, weight circumference, and serum triglycerides.

European Journal of Clinical Nutrition (2010) study showed that vinegar reduces an excess amount of glucose in the blood, when added to a high glycemic index meal (a meal that would normally increase blood glucose).

These studies seem to have one thing in common with each other, improved blood glucose levels. Even though the Japanese study would be indirectly, triglycerides nonetheless have to do with spiked sugar levels and the liver converting this excess glucose to fat.

The one thing I've found in vinegar, that may be a primary factor in controlling blood glucose levels, is chromium. Chromium helps make insulin more effective, by making our cells more sensitive to insulin thus lowering the amount of insulin needed.

If you're diabetic, be careful when adding in apple cider vinegar and start out slow, so adjustments can be made to the amount of insulin taken, (talking to your doctor may be advisable). If you have a problem with hypoglycemia, start out slow so you can make adjustments in your food intake and depending on how severe it is it may be good to talk to your doctor as well.

Appetite control: apple cider vinegar may also have an effect on satiety, according to a study published in the European Journal of Clinical Nutrition (2005), subjects who ate bread with vinegar felt significantly fuller then their counterparts who were fed only bread.

There seems to be a huge amount of benefit in daily consumption of apple cider vinegar, including weight loss through better blood glucose control, and for the price, this daily tonic is hard to beat!

Dosage: start out with 1-2 teaspoons in a cup of water 30-60 minutes prior to each meal and increase it gradually to 2 tablespoons.

Type of apple cider vinegar: the one that is considered the best by many health advocates is raw organic apple cider vinegar with the mother. However, the above research did not have to do with types of apple cider vinegar being better then the other, whether organic, raw or non-organic processed apple cider vinegar. I personally have used both.

If you don't like how it tastes, just think about the powerful health and metabolism boosting effects happening inside your body after you drink it!

The Fat Burning Effect of Food

It may sound crazy, but the foods we select can actually increase the level of thermogenic activity (calorie burning), that happens in our body. This is a big part of why, not all calories are created equal. To say all calories are the same is like saying riding in a car for 5 miles vs. running the 5 miles is the same because the same distance is the same, though they're both the same distance, the one simply burns more calories then the other. This can be the culprit (in problems losing weight) when a person only concerns themselves with a certain number of calories and not where the calories are coming from.

An example of the above would be a salad, several servings of vegetables and a chicken breast vs. a milk shake. The amount of calories you will burn digesting the vegetables (especially raw vegetables) will be much higher then the milk shake. Easy to digest foods jack your sugar levels up and if you're not actively burning this rapid entry of sugar into the blood, it will get carted off to your fatty deposit areas.

1 + 2 = obesity and our current diabetes epidemic:

1. Longer ago, due to less modern conveniences, our ancestors had much more activity in the course of the day, and many of these individuals got much more exercise (from their activities of daily living) then the typical person does today that exercises 3-4 hours per week.

2. Typically an individual or family had 20-50 different food choices or less around them to choose from, (mostly made up of fruits, vegetables, eggs, nuts, meats and dairy) now there are 1000's of fast food, packaged and processed food and snack choices to choose from. Many of these foods almost immediately cause sugar spikes and do not contain the micronutrients that protect us from disease, or the self-regulating fibers that slow down the sugar absorption like natural foods do.

If you add 1 + 2 on a wide spread scale, you have the exact reason we have an obesity and diabetes epidemic. If it was just one and not the other, it wouldn't be so bad, but it isn't, at the same time our choices in food has declined, so has our activity levels. We do not have to figure out where it's coming from or what we need to do, it's as easy as 1 + 2!

The key to creating a fat burning environment: surround yourself with foods that take longer to digest (such as raw vegetables, nuts and other unprocessed foods) and create ways to squeeze in more activity, walking, squatting, taking the stairs, parking further out in the parking lot, rapid house cleaning, yard work or manual labor at your job. You can turn activity into exercise by doing it more rapidly.

The main purpose of eating is calories, but we need those calories to break down over a longer period of time to sustain us properly in keeping our energy levels steady and to avoid sugar spikes as well as the ensuing fatty deposit buildup. When we know the prior meal was heavy, we should always go lighter on our next meal or simply skip the meal.

Example moderate thermic (fat burn) effect: sweet potato (with a little coconut oil and cinnamon), steamed broccoli and tuna. The sweet potato gives carbs that last for quite some time, the fat from the coconut oil gives a long source of energy, the cinnamon gives added sugar control, the tuna gives us good lean protein for building muscle which in turn helps build our metabolism, and the broccoli gives us a great source of fiber and micronutrients. We can substitute beans (black beans, kidney beans etc.) for our meat, or have a little of both.

Example intense thermic effect: salad (oil and vinegar dressing) or other mix of raw vegetables, and grilled chicken or tuna (you can substitute beans for the meat).

Fat burning tool chest for your kitchen: oatmeal, eggs, apples, grapefruit, strawberries, eggs, nuts, berries, broccoli, cauliflower, celery, tomato, beans, quinoa, tuna (grilled fish), grilled chicken.

The above types of foods keep energy levels (blood glucose) steady and shrink fatty deposits!

Two foods that have a negative calorie effect: if a food has a negative calorie effect, it means the food burns more calories then it provides. The two foods that are said to actually burn more calories then they provide are celery and grapefruit.

Burning fat is as easy as 1-2-3:

1. Food choice

2. Activity and exercise

3. Guard your food choices extra much surrounding time periods of low activity.

You cannot put jet fuel into a slow moving vehicle and not expect problems!

Burning Fat Through Brain Power

At the risk of sounding a little over-the-top, I want to discuss the potential of our brain in helping us burn more body fat, lower our body mass index and even lower our blood pressure. When it comes to health and fitness, we often look for things we can add in or take out of our routine, whether it's using fat burners, starting an exercise program, changing our diet etc. And though exercise and changing our diet are two of the most important things we can do, there just may be a powerful tool we're not fully engaging, and that's our brain.

Our body is one of the most powerful producers of personal designer drugs that we can ever hope for, and with the power our brain has, with its signaling system of hormones and nerves throughout the body, I have no doubt it has the capability to increase metabolism, burn more fat and increase muscle gains, when we get a more vivid picture in our mind of what it is we are trying to do, while we're doing it.

Movement burns calories, burns fat, and even builds muscle when we make our muscles work harder then they're used to. So imagine you're burning fat and building muscle whenever you're doing something physical whether in your exercise routine or in your activities of daily living!

This is an abstract from a Harvard University study where some of the participants were made very aware of what they were doing for their health and fitness through manual labor at their jobs.

Abstract: In a study testing whether the relationship between exercise and health is moderated by one's mind-set, 84 female room attendants working in seven different hotels were measured on physiological health variables affected by exercise. Those in the informed condition were told that the work they do (cleaning hotel rooms) is good exercise and satisfies the Surgeon General's recommendations for an active lifestyle. Examples of how their work was exercise were provided. Subjects in the control group were not given this information. Although actual behavior did not change, 4 weeks after the intervention, the informed group perceived themselves to be getting significantly more exercise than before. As a result, compared with the control group, they showed a decrease in weight, blood pressure, body fat, waist-to-hip ratio, and body mass index. These results support the hypothesis that exercise affects health in part or in whole via the placebo effect. PubMed PMID: 17425538

With the obesity problems, as well as heart disease and blood pressure being a looming threat for most of us, the above study should mean a lot! This means, we can change our body composition and even blood pressure, by becoming very aware that our activities of daily living are exercise and that we're burning fat and becoming healthier while we're doing them!

Example: when you exercise or simply do something that increases your level of physical activity), imagine the straining muscles that are turning red with exertion and the fat that is melting down around them to energize and sustain them! Imagine the increased cardio activity going on with your heart, lungs, arteries and veins when you have your heart rate and speed of breathing revved up and then imagine this healthy oxygen and nutrient rich blood flow going to all the parts of the body that you are working.

Have you ever been riding down the road and a song comes on the radio that you haven't heard in a long time that your brain connects up with some long ago memory? Have you felt that tingle go from your head, down your neck and into the rest of your body? Makes you feel like you had the caffeine from several espressos put directly into your veins, right?

The brain is so powerful (that even in this modern era of research capabilities, unlike most of the other parts of our anatomy) we cannot come close to unraveling its complexities, power and capabilities.

Part of the reason I believe in the validity of the above Harvard study, is how easily our brain can trigger a rush of adrenaline and noradrenaline depending on what we encounter, which increases our blood supply as well as our energy and strength levels to the parts of our body that need it. We have a nervous system that revs things up (sympathetic nervous system) and one that calms things down (parasympathetic nervous system). Both can be affected by what we focus on. Should it not make sense, that our capability to burn fat for energy and build muscle would increase, when we become more aware of the benefits of exercise and activity?

Our conscious thought can lead to subconscious reactions throughout our body!

The Fat Burning Effect of Compound Exercises

Compound exercises activate multiple muscle groups and are very effective at incorporating (fat burning, cardio, muscle development and functional strength) into your exercise routine.

My intention was to wrap up the fat burning series in May, but it's hard for me to feel like I finished up properly without including the fat burning effect of compound exercises. Compound movement exercises not only help with strengthening real life movements; they also can help us burn more body fat.

Whether it's bodyweight or added resistance exercises, if you have multiple joints moving it's a compound exercise.

The reason compound exercises can be great cardio: muscle needs blood and oxygen, and working muscles needs a lot of it. The reason our heart rate speeds up and we start breathing faster, is simply to supply blood and oxygen to our working body parts and to carry away the carbon dioxide and other waste products. When we hit our sets back to back by doing alternate exercises for different muscle groups, it keeps this cardio activity peaked.

The reason compound exercises help burn fat: when we keep our heart rate up for an extended time period, (usually for around 20 minutes), it helps trigger the release of body fat for energy; this is what many of us refer to as our 2nd wind.

The reason compound exercises boost the metabolism: our metabolism is largely dependent on how active we are and the amount of toned muscle we have. Toned muscle has a lot more energy consumption and when you have billions of activated muscle cells consuming more calories, your metabolism is going to be higher! When we do resistance (weight bearing, especially free weight) exercises, it builds muscle, thus helping build, maintain and even restore a seemingly old and tired metabolism. A decline in metabolism is not so much aging as it is a loss of muscle.

Going from a pulling to a pushing exercise, lets one muscle group rest while you're doing the next, however your heart and lungs are not getting to rest, and this is why it can turn a muscle building routine into a cardio and fat burning routine as well!

Example: bench pressing and seated row or pushups and bent rows with dumbbells.

Leg exercises such as squats, leg presses, and lunges are great compound exercises for lower body. You can mix a leg exercise in with upper body by doing a pulling exercise, pushing exercise and then a leg exercise, but since legs have so much muscle mass, you can do quite well by working legs by themselves and not resting much between sets.

Try this: get down on the floor and do as many pushups as you can, when you're finished, stand up and do a set of squats. Did you see how your heart rate went up? If this is too hard, lean against a table or into a door opening to do your pushups and hold onto a set of door knobs (or anything that you can steady yourself with) to do your squats.

List of compound exercises: squats, pushups, lunges, rows, shoulder presses, bench presses, deadlifts, power cleans. An intense one is squatting with a set of dumbbells and raising them overhead when coming to a standing position, (cans of food can be used in place of dumbbells).

The neat thing about compound exercises is that they can be done almost anywhere, anytime and are not restricted to when you're in the gym and you do not have to have exercise equipment to benefit from its metabolism boosting effects.

If you want to increase the cardio and fat burning potential of your workout, do a lot of compound movements in the beginning of your routine and keep any of your individual muscle exercises at the end of your routine. This includes things such as biceps curl, triceps push downs, calf exercises, leg extensions. In an exercise routine, compound movements with free weights beats machines hands down due to its activation of stabilizer muscles.

The exercises that facilitate the most muscle during execution, not only helps to burn more fat, it can help increase an athlete's performance, and can help make a senior more mobile!

Sun Fitness

Going into the summer months we all should hope we will get our sun quota and a nice reserve of vitamin D built up (in our fat cells) before going into the fall season and flu season! Isn't it weird how the skin and lotion industry tries to convince us that we should avoid sun exposure by using their chemical laden products?

The sun's ultraviolet light interacts with cholesterol in our skin to make vitamin D and since vitamin D is fat soluble, and can be stored in fat and our liver, this extra vitamin D that we build up during the summer, should help us through the hibernation months of winter. Though it is called a vitamin, vitamin D is actually a hormone and a body's shortage of this hormone has been linked to most chronic diseases we have today, and most of us know that hormonal imbalances can get a lot of things off track!

Our body was designed to interact in a positive way with the sun and with regular exposure; this can be one of nature's greatest gifts to our health! And with all the benefits it gives us, if our children got more of it, they probably would have immune systems more prepared to overcome the exposures when they start back to school.

We are advised now to use sunscreens for any part of our body not covered with clothes, anytime we're exposed to the sun, whether it's between the house and the car, our drive to work, or even if we have a window in our office. Can you imagine how much sunblock could get used throughout the world, if everyone in it starts using sun block lotions?

EVERYTHING on this planet would die without the sun, and when organizations like these advocate toxic sunscreens (for any exposure someone may possibly have to it), we should place no value in them or their advocacy of the companies they fail to tell us that they actually represent. They are no different then lobbyists sent from the corporate dairy industry (cloaked as our U.S.D.A.) to convince lawmakers that raw milk is dangerous for our health. Either one has been around for thousands of years longer then these industry fear mongers or lawmakers and (if the world doesn't end) my guess is, the health benefits of either will still be undeniable long after they're gone.

 These advocacy groups do not bother telling us (during their skin care and sunblock promo speeches) that Octyl Methoxycinnamate has been shown to be toxic, but still is in 90% of the sunscreens and has been shown to be particularly toxic when exposed to sunshine.

 Most of us already know, that too much of a good thing can be bad, and the sun is no different. Sunburn causes inflammation and chronic inflammation can lead to cancer of the skin. When we suddenly expose skin (that isn't used to being in the sun) to several hours' exposure, we are asking for problems.

Sun exposure is really no different then exercise, (even though it's healthy) too much exercise can lead to inflammation of the joints and continued inflammation can lead to chronic diseased joint conditions. Chronic inflammation of our skin can lead to skin cancer.

Disclaimer: if I was in a situation where I was suddenly out in the sun for hours, and my skin was not conditioned for it and I had no good way of covering up, I would probably use whatever sunblock happens to be available, but I would only be doing it for protection from sunburn and not protection from the sun. The sun is good, sunburns are bad and the sooner we can figure that out, the better off we'll be!

Foods good for skin color: vitamin A rich foods are really good for healthy skin color, orange foods such as cantaloupe, sweet potatoes, orange and yellow peppers and apricots.

Foods good for skin protection: colorful compounds (carotenoids) from fruits and vegetables get deposited in the skin and protect us against sunburn and aging (oxidation) of the skin. These pigments and colors in plant life use the sun to build food, and have their purpose in giving our skin good synergy with the sun as well.

Sunburn remedies: soak a clean towel in apple cider vinegar and lay it over the affected area, it will instantly soothe your skin and help the burn heal faster. You can also get in a tub of water, getting it as hot as you can, until you break a sweat; this will help release the heat that is trapped under your skin and help your skin break its fever.

Regular skin exposure to the sun is like regular activity to muscle, it's healthy for it.

Pumping Up the Flab!

 Many of us bring in a New Year with ambitious goals to shed body fat before summer and often renew that commitment when we start feeling hints of spring in the air. Oft times we feel that we have let ourselves and our fitness goals down when we feel the hot summer breezes blowing...

 Because the industry is so weight loss driven, we primarily think of ways to burn more body fat, but what about the empty void (the flab)? What about the remaining fat that has very little muscle under it? Why is it that even some thin people can appear saggy and flabby? Have you ever noticed how some people look really good at a heavier weight? We hear the term pleasantly plump, but whether skinny or fat, we never hear the expression, "pleasantly flabby!"

There are 3 things that give our body its shape:

1. Bones

2. Muscle

3. Fat

And of course our skin stretched out nicely overtop of our fat, muscle and bones, helps make it look nice most of the time.

Fat with muscle pumped up under it actually can give a person a very healthy look and is one of the best short cuts for getting shaped up quickly! There are approximately 3500 calories in a pound of fat so it takes quite a bit of daily calorie deficits to make a noticeable difference, but it doesn't take long at all to tone and pump untoned muscle back into its prior conditioning.

Muscle shrinks or gains size according to how it gets used and it regains its prior conditioning very rapidly and most adults (that have gotten flabby) have quite a bit of mature muscle that is simply waiting on the signal to regain its size. Whether it's under body fat or under skin that seems saggy and loose, this added muscle can rapidly change your shape!

How to do it: do exercises for all parts of the body, but then specifically target the body parts that bother you the most, with exercises that build muscle in these areas. You can get a series of exercises for these areas by going online and ask for the best exercises for this area, such as "best exercises for shoulders," "best exercises for legs," and "best exercises for the core."

Muscle pumping tips...

Shoulders: most overhead shoulder presses with dumbbells or bar.

Back: most rowing exercises, lat pull-down and chin-ups.

Chest: most pressing movements, such as bench presses and pushups.

Back of the arms (triceps): this part of our arms gets flabby because we don't use our pushing muscles as much as our pulling muscles. You can do pushups against a table or other raised surface if you can't do regular pushups. It really targets triceps if you put your hands close together.

Legs: squats, lunges and deadlifts.

Buttocks: if you're trying to tone the buttocks, (do the leg exercises listed above), but push with your heels, this transfers the resistance away from your knees and quadriceps and puts the added resistance in your hamstrings and buttocks.

Example: if you're doing squats at home you can hold onto something and lean backwards until most of your weight is on your heels, (slightly pick up the front of your feet) then drop down into as low a squat as you can, only using the object you're holding on to, for support. You can also put a mat or book under your heel when doing freestanding squats. If you're doing smith machine squats, position feet further out in front of you. If you're using a leg press, put your feet higher on the platform and push with your heels.

 Tip: remember you're trying to pump tone into your sagging body part, so you do not want to rest long between sets as this causes you to lose the toning and pumping effect. Go as heavy as you can for about 12 reps and only rest for 30-60 seconds between sets. If you are using your body weight for your exercises such as squats, lunges and pushups, increasing the speed, increases the resistance.

Flabbiness and a loss of shape, mostly comes from a lack of muscle. Adding more muscle gives us a better shape, strengthens our bones, protects our joints and makes our activities of daily living become easier!

Human Radiator

Definition of radiator: an engine cooling device in a motor vehicle or aircraft consisting of a bank of thin tubes in which circulating fluid is cooled by the surrounding air.

Human radiator: when we get warm, our body increases the blood flow outwards toward the skin so we can push out the excess heat through sweat and gasses. We have over 50,000 miles of arteries, arterioles and capillaries, so this system is a powerful one at pushing excess heat out of our body!

Our thermostat: the hypothalamus helps us keep our temperature within a tight range whether we need to warm up or cool down due to our activities (both internal and external) and our surrounding environment. A lot of this is handled by it switching primary directions of blood flow.

Our brain gets 20% of our blood flow, so it can easily detect an increase or decrease in temperature (in the hypothalamus) and it has mechanisms it uses to change direction of blood flow (shunting) as well as a capability to increase or decrease urine concentration to keep our blood volume steady.

There are some ways we can help keep this cooling system from getting overloaded and help prevent heat stroke and heat related fatigue...

Opening the air ducts: one of the best ways to help our body get rid of heat is to not wear clothes that hold the heat in, this is good in cold weather but not good if you're trying to help your body with its cooling efforts. Anything we can do to cool the skin helps, especially areas that have a lot of blood flow.

Keeping our radiator full: if we do not stay hydrated our blood volume will shrink, making it harder for our body to push the heat out to the skin for release through sweat and gasses. If your heart rate starts increasing (even though your work output has not) chances are that your fluid levels are getting low.

Cold water: drinking cold water is a good way to help ease the workload on our body's cooling system. Just like a warm drink helps warm our body when it's cold, cold water helps cool the body down. And because of the physiological effects of cold water in the body, it should be a source of energy on a hot day!

Electrolytes: sodium, potassium, magnesium, calcium and chloride are very important electrolytes for maintaining fluid balance as well as many things that help our body function properly, and should be gotten primarily through a balanced diet. However, using an occasional electrolyte supplement (such as a sports drink or electrolyte powder/tablet) for times that you sweat a lot can be a good way to maintain a healthy fluid balance. I personally like the powder or tablet electrolytes over sport drinks, since most sports drinks have the unhealthy downside of additives that enhance taste but have little or nothing to do with electrolyte balance.

 Food: the type of food we eat can make a BIG difference in how we handle summer heat. Digestion takes a lot of blood and when we eat heavy, high fat/protein foods (that require more digestive energy), it makes us feel bad because of the body shunting blood flow away from the digestive tract to push excess heat out of our skin. These heavy foods will sit in our system like a block of wood until we cool off and blood can return to aid in digestion.

Note: fruits are a great food to eat when you have to be out in the heat.

Example: watermelon is cooling, has high water content, is rich in potassium, has a considerable amount of calcium and magnesium, (add a little salt) and you have a pretty tasty source of electrolytes!

 Our body has powerful capabilities of heating and cooling itself, but we can do some things that make its job much easier and when we do this, it can put the energy saved toward giving us more energy for doing the things we have to do!

Tummy Flattening Effect of Fiber

One of the fastest ways to flatten our abdominal area is to eat a fiber rich diet, and I'm not referring to a cereal loaded diet, (most cereals spike blood sugar) but rather a diet that has lots of raw vegetables, beans, oatmeal, nuts and fruit in it.

Insoluble fiber is like a slow moving bulldozer to the waste inside our colon. When we have a daily diet rich in fiber, it works a lot like a street sweeper that keeps the street and gutters clear of debris.

It's not unusual (with the typical American diet) for individuals to carry 5-20 pounds of waste in their colon and this can cause the abdominal area to protrude.

Clearing the colon is much more important initially then fat loss, because of the dangers associated with a colon that is filled with old toxic waste. The best way to deal with potential colon cancer is a change of diet, along with regular activity and exercise (to stimulate bowel movements), not a series of diagnostics, surgeries and chemotherapy!

Example of why food sticks in our gut: we have a tendency to eat fries and bread buns with our meat instead of broccoli and beans like we used to 50-60 years ago. Have you ever noticed that after thousands of years, foods that were considered a staple in a person's diet suddenly becomes prime suspect in digestive tract issues? This is about as ignorant as blaming a highway for a traveler's flat tires instead of the nails that were on it.

One of the first steps for weight loss should be to clear the colon, (this helps clear the path for getting rid of toxins associated with weight loss). To do this, a good colon cleanse really helps kick things off. After this initial cleanse, a fiber rich diet will not only help keep the colon clear of old waste, but will help prevent colon cancer as well.

Cleansing phase: for 7 days switch to a diet almost completely made up of raw or lightly steamed vegetables, fruits, nuts, beans and oatmeal with some added fats, such as fish oil, coconut oil and olive oil. Drink plenty of water to stay hydrated and for flushing toxins out. This cleansing phase can get a little tough, so you really want to keep it strong in your mind what it is you are doing this for. Keep some raw local grown honey around to use for an energy booster. Drinking cold water can help boost energy levels and boost metabolism. Adding in a fiber supplement or a good detox program can boost results.

Maintenance phase: should be a diet with plenty of raw fruits, vegetables, nuts, and beans mixed in. These foods help move other foods in our diet along and help prevent build up. If you have gut health and bowel movement issues, I highly recommend using a fiber supplement and adding in enzymes. Try to eat foods that have 3-5 grams of fiber per serving, this helps keep our blood sugar from spiking, helps lower cholesterol, and keeps us regular and our waistline trim!

A diet rich in fiber helps prevent a buildup of waste in our waist!

Questions on Pills, Guns and False Flags

I'm not a brain specialist, psychologist, media or political analyst but I do have a few questions...

Who benefits from several 100 million people being riled up with angst among themselves, it doesn't seem to be you and I...so who does?

Why at this particular time in history, (while our government is still claiming that terrorism and world unrest is abounding), is this same government constantly on a campaign to unarm its citizens, (every single time something happens) when an armed populace should be a well meaning government's greatest ally and defender of the homeland?

Is the recent movement by the Supreme Court of the United States (SCOTUS) to allow gay marriage, followed with the gay flag beamed on the White House and the sudden jumping through hoops of corporations to remove anything pertaining to the rebel flag, from TV shows, Nascar (and now Bubba Watson and the General Lee) a show of how much they care, or is it simply a demonstration of a central (Federal) government's choking power hold over individual states rights to choose? Why is a flag being appropriate or not a question for today instead of 150 years ago? If it represents the wrongful era of slavery, should it not have been put in a museum after the Democrats lost their war for slavery 150 years ago?

 Could all these events, simply be to get people's attention off of the angst our leaders are creating abroad, and instead keep our focus on the differences we have among us, until we get the cold bucket of water slapped in our face of their real intent with our country?

 Why do we not hear a little more about who raised Dylan Roof and who influenced the final molding of this hateful, person, who would set in a church with unarmed individuals whom he killed in return for their hospitality? Why is the total focus being put into tying this heinous act, to a flag and guns? Isn't this ignorant to cast blame on external objects for something that was quite obviously happening internally in this young man's brain by the hate that he demonstrated? After all is the wrapper dangerous or is it the poison inside that can cause harm?

Why don't we hear more about the prescription history of these deranged individuals (such as this one) that go in and shoot up unarmed and defenseless people? Why does the media not cover the fact of what has changed in mental health and the fact that most of these killers have two things in common, doing their crime amongst people who are the least likely to be armed and a history of selective serotonin re-uptake inhibitors, (S.S.R.I.) pharmaceutical drug use?

Why is it that the United States is the largest prisoner of its own population, largely due to its war on drugs, but is the largest legal drug dealer and consumer in the world? Isn't this like saying, "you gotta be my-kind-of-wrong to be right?"

Selective serotonin re-uptake inhibitors (S.S.R.I. drug) use has grown in popularity in anything from modifying children's behavior (good behavior in a pill) to helping adults to not care about depressing situations. Is this a good idea or is this like a borderline diabetic that chooses to be on insulin instead of making lifestyle changes?

If something changes the way you or your child's brain processes information, isn't it like rewiring the brain? If a psychopath's brain were put in your head, would you still be you, or would you be the psychopath? If the new brain changed the actions you took with your body, would it not be 100% due to the fact that you have a brain that processes things differently in your head? How much control do you have over your body's actions when your brain suddenly perceives things in a different way? Likewise when a brain gets dependent on a chemical for processing external things in a positive manner, what happens when the person suddenly stops taking the drug, and they have a brain that goes bat-crazy?

Disclaimer: I believe there are times some of these drugs may be the best answer for chemical imbalances, but should this not be reserved for the most extreme cases instead of a broad base prescription model that puts industry profits ahead of a country's mental health?

False fear and confusion flags are for the purpose of diverting attention from the real thing, and one thing our government, media and pharmaceutical industry seem to all have in common, is their constant diversion of attention away from the underlying cause of the problems, and their appreciation for a good false flag to further their own agenda.

We Weigh Too Much Because We...

Quite simply, the reason Americans on average weigh too much, is because we eat way too much! It's no telling how many billions of tons of food calories Americans have stored up in the form of body fat. A period of famine certainly wouldn't kill nearly as many people in America as it would in some other countries and according to research (on caloric restriction), just might extend life. As responsible individuals and good stewards of the world we live in, we really should become more need driven and a lot less pleasure driven with our fuel intake. This would take a huge burden off our food and our healthcare systems.

There are many reasons we excuse weight gain, whether it's a slowing of metabolism, thyroid problems, or not having access to the right foods. For the most part however, our weight problems simply come from over consumption of easy to digest calories and too little activity to burn them off.

When we constantly take in foods that are low in fiber (most processed snack foods, breads, pastas and other primarily starch foods) it keeps our glucose/ blood sugar levels and insulin in our blood too high and this shuts off our capability to burn body fat.

When we have excess body fat and we have a low activity day ahead of us, it does not hurt us at all, to sometimes simply skip eating for 18-24 hours. Many people that know me know that I like to do the intermittent fasting (IF) or very low calories on my non-workout days. I figure this is a good day for me to skip eating, (since my calorie needs are much less). This causes my body to pull the calories it needs from stored fat. I've gotten to where I enjoy this way of keeping my bodyweight under control and once I get past the sugar low (around 12:00 pm for me), it's really not that bad.

We often think we have to have sugar when our energy runs low, but we need to do is wait a little longer to let the circulating insulin drop, then our body will start releasing its stored energy. And you can definitely trust the fact that your body knows how to access calories from its own snack machine (stored fat) when it isn't getting calories from our digestive tract!

How food ages us: food is something we need to sustain life, but it also has a direct impact on aging and when we have a constant over consumption of food, we simply age our body faster. Our digestive processes produce free radicals and free radicals produce oxidation. Oxidation is a root cause of pre-mature aging and chronic disease, and this excess oxidation is like the smoke that doesn't get expelled from a factory that is processing more then it should. In much the same way, when we constantly eat more then our body needs to be processing, we'll simply age faster.

One of the best things we can do for weight loss, (or avoiding weight gain) is to watch our sugar and starch intake when we are going to be fairly inactive. When we have this excess sugar in our blood, insulin will be produced to remove the excess, (the insulin does not burn the excess sugar, it stores it). And until the insulin has done its job and leaves the blood, our fat burning mechanisms get turned off! This doesn't apply so much to eating sugars prior to really being active, or right after a lot of activity, (these are the times your body will suck it up for energy). So to keep your body in fat burn mode, lowering your intake of sugars and starches during low output time periods and increasing it when there is high energy output.

 The fat burning fire is lot like a bonfire, the right amount of fuel will keep it blazing, but if you dump too much on it, the flame will be smothered and it will take it a while to fire back up!

The One Cancer Doctor
Who Got Caught

Many of us probably heard about the popular oncologist (cancer doctor) in Michigan and the $35 million dollar chemotherapy fraud.

His charges: deliberate misdiagnosis of patients as having cancer, giving unnecessary chemotherapy, even to end of life patients who will not benefit.

Chemotherapy is a carcinogen and CARCINOGENS CAUSE CANCER! According to the charges, his doctor was deliberately poisoning people and very likely will be THE root cause for many of his patient's cancer!

Our bodies fight cancer every single day on its own and to put our faith in a poison industry (oncologists) to control our cancers is about as risky as hiring a thief to guard our property. It has gotten more and more that going to a medical facility will yield a diagnosis for a condition that will qualifying you for continuing care, whether it's to be on pharmaceutical drug treatments or a continuing onslaught of doctor's office visits and diagnostic procedures in their witch hunt to find something.

The cancer industry has gotten huge and powerful and its need for more patients has grown in lockstep. If there ever were a cure (other then healthy lifestyle changes), the ones that built this industry would see their lucrative money machine implode. With all the pharmaceutical drug incentives for long term care, for us not to not think the temptation is there to over-diagnose, is like walking onto a car lot and asking the sales person if he or she thinks you need a car.

Cancer most times comes from stem cells that produce organ tissue. When carcinogens (toxins) are not gotten rid of properly it can mess up the blueprint for the next generation of cells, (whether it's how they're shaped or how they look). The stem cell is the mold for our new replacement cells.

Example: if a mold used to manufacture rubber tires got bent, it could effect the shape of the tire produced as well as the way the tire behaves and if we get lumpy, weak tires on our vehicle, it can effect how the vehicle operates and potentially cause the vehicle to get totaled. The cancer industry has created an entire business model on trying to repair millions of tires instead of the mold that is producing the miss-shaped tires.

We need healthy stem cells to produce new cells for revitalization of our body parts, but when these cells get produced in an abnormal fashion it can eventually get in the way or how the organ functions. These cells can also drift away from their original organ and attach and grow somewhere else in the body. This is why cancers are named after the place they originated from.

Environmental toxins and bad lifestyle habits are the leading causes of messing up our stem cell's blueprint for how they're supposed to produce new cells, (whether its brain cells, liver cells, pancreatic cells, kidney cells, bones cells, lung cells, skin cells etc.).

When an organ or body part is already hurting and we elect to do a biopsy, surgery, radiation or chemotherapy poisoning of this body part or organ, we are using a top down approach that can be more hurtful and harmful then doing absolutely nothing except changes in lifestyle that address the root cause.

3 Cancerous questions about Chemo, Radiation and Surgery:

1. Chemotherapy is carcinogenic and carcinogens cause cancer, so even if it shrinks the cancer, does it not increase the chance of us getting cancer somewhere else?

2. Radiation messes up cell structure, but isn't cancer actually caused by cells that get messed up and then go on to reproduce screwed up generations of cells that eventually turn into screwed up lumps of tissue that later get diagnosed as cancer?

3. Surgery is to remove the obvious lump of cancer but it doesn't get rid of the stem cell that is producing the cancer, so isn't this like cutting blight off of a plant leaf and acting like the plant is free of the blight?

Dr. Farid Fata's gave unnecessary treatments to 533 patients, how many of them were healthy people who simply gave into cancer industry fear mongering (that gets even the healthy to go in for cancer screenings)? There are a lot of incentives to prescribing pharmaceuticals and keeping diagnostic machines occupied, so how often is this happening in a country that has its population on more drugs (that are legal) then any country on this planet? Given the 5-year survival statistics, what percentage of cancer patients would've been much better off with their cancer left undiscovered?

One of the first things a farmer does, if an area of his farm has problems is to do an analysis of the soil to check for deficiencies, (by doing this, he can restore this area back to health and bring it back up to par with the rest of his farm. Should I not check the soil around myself that might be feeding or shrinking the cancers that are attempting to develop.

The soil is: air, water, food, exercise and activity, sunshine, rest and sleep, positive family, social and community connections as well as a strong faith in the Master Healer.

The Human Cell Tower and Its Cellular Language

Long before there were cell towers, cell phones and satellites, there were human cell towers, each one with several trillion surrounding cells, listening and then behaving according to the information they receive from their cell tower.

We have the capability to send out strong or weak signals to the cells of our body, by the lifestyle choices we make every day.

Example: when someone calls us over a cellular device and their voice comes through crystal clear, it makes so we can respond in a clear and precise manner to the information received and react accordingly. The cells of our body respond in much the same way when they receive their signals from a cell tower that has cleaned up its lifestyle habits and can send out clear, healthy and strong signals for building the next generation of cells.

We reproduce billions of cells every day, (this is what helps us grow and what keeps us rejuvenated). When our cells receive an unclear signal from us, (because of unhealthy lifestyle habits) they have the potential of producing weird shaped cells that have the potential to misbehave in our body. These are the things that produce chronic diseases such as cancer.

Example: imagine a fleet of 1000 employees surrounding a worksite, all relying on information received through a nearby cell tower, each employee receives his or her message crystal clear and each one knows precisely how to do their job. Things would function and flow smoothly right? Now imagine the tower gets neglected and run down because the operator decides the simple basic rules of maintenance are not necessary. It may start out with only a few problems and communication errors, but gradually the capability to communicate effectively diminishes, and quite predictably, the surrounding fleet of 1000 employees is unable to get information to do their jobs properly and chaos starts to breakout!

Projects are not finished, and the products that are made are not designed according to the original blueprint and if changes are not made soon enough, the worksite will close down due to all the malfunctions.

To remedy problems, we should not spend our time looking at symptoms, but rather what is causing the symptom. Why would we get prescribed a medicine for a bellyache when we could stop eating the food that gives us the bellyache or digestive problems?

Something that really intrigues me is how different types of food cause certain reactions in our body, (this is why a balanced diet works so well). There are foods that give us energy, there are foods that help us rebuild, and there are foods that help us fight disease. When we combine these with the other healthy lifestyle basics, it helps us to detox, build, repair and energize our body and will send out a clear signal to build a healthy or healthier generation of cells.

It is a big mistake to think we can constantly breathe in toxins, eat and drink junk food, lead inactive lives, stay under stress, not get our rest, and still produce health and not disease.

We have the opportunity to speak health to the cells of our body through our healthy habits and the way we think and believe. The stronger and more positive we make these 3, the stronger the signal will be from our cell tower!

1 million seconds is 13 days, 1 billion seconds is 31 years, 1 trillion seconds is 31,688 years, you are made up of several trillion cells. Our body produces on average about 10 billion cells a day.

Our habits send out signals 24 hours a day, 7days a week, 365 days a year to the several trillion cells in our body, whether for wellness or disease...

Gym of Your Future!

Our main concern in fitness should be that it prepares us in advance for the capabilities or the conditioning we want for our future. If we want to prepare our body to have a lot of sitting in our future, all we have to do is a lot of setting around, and we can assure ourselves of a future of sitting on our keister as well as placing the demand for assistance with our activities of daily living (ADL's) on other people!

Over the past 20-30 years, (like most other things) technology has advanced exercise equipment and many other widgets and apps that are the latest and greatest breakthrough in health and fitness. The hype that is behind some of these ads is almost enough to make someone feel like they're getting in shape just reading or listening to all the things it claims it will do!

Whether it's our sources of food, reduction in body fat or exercise, we have become mentally conditioned to constantly look for and then to buy into things that make health and fitness easier, but there are NO REAL shortcuts when it comes to health and fitness. A change of lifestyle is the real anecdote for getting in shape, getting rid of chronic disease in the body and for building optimal health and wellness! Keeping it basic, simple, and cheap is the best way to avoid the financial and gimmick pitfalls. The top 2 things that would address most people's health and fitness concerns can be summed up in one sentence; less (but more nutritious) food, and regular challenging activities.

The Gym of Your Future: what I like to call the futuristic gym, is your life and is simply doing activities today that you want to be able to do tomorrow, next week, or next month. In other words, if you want to be able to walk the trail with your family at a weekend camping trip, don't use the motor scooter in the grocery store, (let someone that really needs it, use it). We cannot expect to get people around us (as well as gadgets of convenience) to do all our physical work without our own physical capabilities shrinking in the process. Our immune system is the same, if we do not expose ourselves to our surroundings, our immune system will get weak, and unable to protect us from our surroundings.

Gap fillers: exercise sessions are gap fillers for a lifestyle that doesn't provide enough physical activity for the level of fitness (or amount of muscularity) a person wants, just as supplements are gap fillers for diets that are lacking in certain nutrients. The above two can add value into a person's life, but I believe it's important that they are looked at as gap fillers.

Gap filler clause: we should all be conditioned to handle more then our daily routine requires of us, life has a way of handing us the unexpected. And exercise is one of the best ways to condition ourselves to better handle whatever it is we have to do in our daily lives, no matter if you're a world class athlete or a senior that simply wants to stay independent and not reliant on others for daily living.

Whenever we have the opportunity at home, or work to do physical activity or manual labor, we should look at it as a muscle and fitness building opportunity. These are the real life exercises that help prevent injury when we attempt to do it tomorrow, next week and next year!

Your activities today are tomorrow's physical capability insurance!

How Negatives and Injuries Strengthen Us

The way our body gains strength and muscle is one of the more intriguing sides of health and fitness to me. We have a tendency of taking the path of least resistance, when oft times this is the very thing that will build us up.

Muscle and strength are built through injury from doing something the muscle isn't used to doing, the body simply responds by rebuilding the muscle bigger, faster and stronger so that it can handle the new stress better.

Our muscles also respond in exactly the opposite way when we avoid physical stress, by shrinking and weakening muscle, (muscle atrophy). An increase or a decrease in muscle tone, size, strength and capabilities (through our action or inaction) is simply our body doing what we tell it to do.

Positives and Negatives: when we do a set of arm curls, 1 repetition would be the curl upward and the lowering of the bar back to the start position. The positive part of the movement is the curling upward, the negative is the lowering back down to the start position. **Positive** = the lifting part of the movement, **Negative** = the lowering part of the movement.

What stands out to me in this whole muscle building process is how the least impressive part of a repetition (the negative) is the most responsible for growth. Injury stimulates the need for new muscle growth and negatives cause the greatest injury to muscle tissue.

Example: when we do a bench press, it's hard to impress ourselves and the others around us by the control we exhibit in lowering the bar to our chest, so most of the attention is put in the thrust upward. However, when we lower the bar and weights rapidly, and then bounce off the chest, to help us drive the bar upward in the positive part of the movement, (we are depriving ourselves of a very powerful stimulator of muscle strength and growth)!

Using good form in exercise not only helps protect us from the injuries and muscle imbalances that using bad form can bring, it is also a major stimulator in muscle building, strengthening and toning!

What helps me the most to know what is good form, is to know the 2 primary contributing factors in muscle building and strengthening.

The 2 main contributing factors are: muscle stretch and muscle tension. Most times the stretch is going to be felt during the negative part of the movement and the tension felt in the positive part of the movement. The negative part of the movement should be done slower and the positive should be done faster.

The human body is designed to use stress and injury as signaling mechanisms to stimulate an increase in strength, whether it's mental or physical. If we avoid physical or mental stress, our corresponding systems will get weaker and weaker. Keeping ourselves challenged both mentally and physically is important if we are to keep or improve what we've been blessed with.

I had something happen here at the gym yesterday, that put me through probably the worst work project that I've had in the past 10 years, but weird thing is, I'm happier since then and everything in my life seems easier! So obviously (at least for me), negatives and adversity help both physically and mentally.

The positive things in life look and feel great, but how we handle the negatives and recover from our injuries, plays a big part in building true strength, endurance and character!!

Personal Designer Drugs
Your Body Makes

The body's capability to produce its own drugs is one of the most amazing things to me about the human body. It makes antibodies, and other chemicals produced by the immune system, as well as brain drugs, drugs that break things down, drugs that build things up, drugs that make us happy etc. We can certainly trust the fact that we have an internal pharmacy that is at work 24 hours a day, 7 days a week, 365 days a year!

We have many pharmaceutical drugs available (that work very well at speeding things up), but it's our own body in the end that gets rid of things, balances things out and heals things that have gotten off track.

Example: there are things that have no business being in our body and are considered foreign invaders. Our body will produce antibodies (anti-body) that are specifically designed for the type of infection, illness etc. that we have.

We use these anti-bodies as a tagging system to mark the foreign invaders (that are in our body) for destruction. We have a messaging system that gathers the information on the invader, (whether it's a cancer or a flu-bug), it will then deliver this information to the immune system. The immune system will then start rapidly formulating drugs that are specifically designed for this foreign invader. The antibodies have meanwhile tagged and flagged the bad things for destruction by our immune system.

Our immune system is so powerful that if it over-reacts it can kill the entire body rapidly (such as in anaphylactic shock). Fortunately our body has a messaging system that (if working properly) signals the exact amount of force that is needed to destroy the things that do not belong in our body.

Example: if you take care of your house, you will know exactly what does and what does not belong in your home, whether it's something that is no longer of value, or something that came in from the outside such as dirt, bugs, trash, etc. If you go through the house and tag these things that are of no value and create a bad environment, the cleanup crew will know exactly what to remove and destroy because these items are marked for destruction and are considered (anti-home). Antibiotics work in much the same way and are simply drugs that are produced by the body to tag the bad stuff so the chemicals from our immune system can kill and remove them.

There are things we can do such as getting external assistance (from a doctor, surgeon or pharmaceutical drug), to correct things and to speed things up, but it is very important that we know that it is our body that has the lone responsibility of healing itself, how we strengthen or weaken this system is largely up to us.

There are many chemical reactions that are produced in the body, and though it has a very complicated process, what these processes rely on is very basic and not complicated at all!

These are the basic ingredients our internal laboratory (immune system) uses to make drugs designed specifically for our needs, these were the same 1000's of years ago and they're still the same today:

1. Clean air, (oxygen).

2. Hydration (water).

3. Healthy diet.

4. Active lifestyle and exercise.

5. Sunshine.

6. Deep rest and recovery.

7. Positive social connections (family, friends, community).

When you do the above with consistency, your body not only produces drugs designed specifically for you and the bad things your body is fighting every day such as cancer, heart disease, stress etc. it also produces the chemicals that help increase energy, vitality and happiness! God designed something unmatchable when he designed our body's chemistry...

For thou didst form my inward parts: Thou didst cover me in my mother's womb. I will give thanks unto thee, for I am fearfully and wonderfully made~ Psalm 139, 13-14

A Fountain of Violence They Won't Admit To

August 26, 2015: the airwaves were covered by the horrendous shootings of a reporter and cameraman in Roanoke, VA. And once again things are being shaped to divert attention away from one simple thing that has changed in the past 30 years. You will hear anything from "we need stricter gun laws," to "we need more mental health assistance for these individuals," to one of the parents saying that "if necessary he'll become the John Walsh of gun control." However, you will not hear a single reporter, interviewee or news anchor say..."PULL THIS NUT JOB'S PAST & PRESENT PRESCRIPTION HISTORY!" That's the diagnosis they should look at plain and simple, but they don't want to look at the fountain from which spews their never ending news stories and their advertiser's revenue sources do they? They have their willing partner, (the Federal government) which is a willing partner since enhanced gun laws help fulfill a dictatorial agenda.

 For just once I would like to hear the powers that be address what is causing all these intense bouts of mental illness. I would like to hear them admit, they are trying to tighten gun control because of the mistakes they made in broad spread, uncontrolled, S.S.R.I. usage and that they simply want to clear the path for Big Pharma and their political cronies to be able to continue to make the same profitable mistakes on a trusting populace.

 If we do not take a serious look at what brain drugs are doing to our future mental health, we are going to continue having horrific things happen as has happened in Aurora, Colorado (James Holmes), Charleston, South Carolina (Dylann Roof), and Roanoke, Virginia (Bryce Williams). I see this struggle as being directly at the top between drug companies, and the NRA. Drug companies and their policy cronies want to create a safe path for the drugs they create and the NRA wants to keep the road paved for the ones they represent. My belief is neither one actually represents you and I.

I am not a psychologist but a lot of my life has been spent studying health, fitness, and chronic disease prevention as well as cause and effect. And one thing that you should go after like a laser is the cause, not the effect. When a person in a trusted position of authority uses a top down approach (by addressing effects and not causes) they are either uneducated or have an agenda.

If we don't acknowledge and change the things we are doing that are wrongfully shaping our children's future and make the changes we need to now, this problem is going to grow like a cancer lump being fed a steady stream of pure sugar.

If a person gets on these S.S.R.I. drugs to help them suppress emotions, what happens if the conscious is suppressed...it's an emotion as well? It may feel good to a person to "just not care," but how does it affect the ones that have to deal with this person? What happens if they suddenly get off the drug and their brain is as one on fire? When we have a massive amount of people on these drugs and an industry that is constantly pressing for even more expanded usage, what we will have left is a conscious suppressed generation of drug induced sociopaths that are like potential time bombs.

We have a conscious mind that is supposed to bother us, depress us and guide us to help us to make things better for ourselves and the ones we care about, so should we be throwing pills down our throat that tell our brains to chemically alter itself so as to not care or to feel differently about these things?

Example: the Paxil Defense has been established in court, and has been used successfully as a defense in crimes due to lack of self control when the crime occurred. This has also been used for other S.S.R.I.'s including Wellbutrin and Zoloft. Please checkout the S.AV.E. Project www.thesaveproject.com, to see the common link (many violent offenders have with each other) that the media is not talking about.

These drugs have very addictive effects as well, if you do not believe it, watch how someone's behavior changes that suddenly quits. The medical industry however does not use addiction as a terminology for this; they call it "discontinuation syndrome."

This is our and our children's future and if we let the pharmaceutical industry grow the use of these drugs in our life and that of our children we will be sitting on a ticking time bomb of tragedies like this.

Roanoke, VA is where my dad, brother and I were hospitalized after our plane crash in Virginia, so this latest tragedy struck home a little harder. And I really hope the tragedy that hit Roanoke will not be dishonored by using it to further agendas (that are fed strictly by effects) and that absolutely do nothing to address the actual causes.

Whether an ax, sword, hammer, vehicle or gun is used in a violent act on oneself or someone else, this violence has a source and the demonization of the object is about as ignorant as a person that is upset from continually having to mop up water on a floor, when they themselves refuse to acknowledge and turn off the faucet...But then there happens to be no profit in slowing down the distribution of S.S.R.I. drugs is there?

What would happen if only psychiatrists would be allowed to distribute these drugs? My guess is there would be an unacceptable amount of drug dealers for an industry that is responsible for the REAL drug problem in America...

Controlling Blood Sugar With...

 Have you ever paid attention to some of the ads for drugs that help control blood sugar? Have you noticed the short amount of time that is spent on the list of benefits, with the majority spent on warnings about side effects and potential side effects? There is one that is being advertised now (Invokana/canagliflozin) that has a list of 43 potential side effects.

 Would it not be better for our body, to simply quit eating foods that spike our blood sugar? Would it not be better to avoid sweet foods when it isn't just before or right after periods of intense activity? Does it not make sense to control blood sugar through our diet (given the fact that sugars are much more the problem in causing cholesterol and fatty deposits then the fat in our diet)?

 Excerpt from Dr. Osborne: Diabetes is an epidemic in the US. The condition can cause obesity, kidney damage, blindness, loss of limb, neuropathy, and much more. Unfortunately most doctors deal with this condition like this: "Mrs. Jones, your blood sugar levels are high. I am going to prescribe you a medication to help you control them. I will need you to watch your diet closely. Limit your sugar intake; eat plenty of whole grains and vegetables. You will also need to exercise more. Because diabetes runs in your family, you will probably need to take this medication for the rest of your life. In addition, to this medicine, I am going to also prescribe you a statin to ensure that your cholesterol stays low. Studies show that managing cholesterol aggressively helps with people who have blood sugar problems." You see, the drugs don't fix the problem, they only mask the diabetic condition while silently wrecking your nutritional status~ Dr. Peter Osborne is a Chiropractor and Board Certified doctor of clinical nutrition in Sugar Land, Texas.

 This epidemic of Type 2 Diabetes is primarily caused by the types of food that we eat and low levels of activity to burn off the resulting blood sugar spikes. These constant spikes in blood sugar lead to insulin resistance and when our trillions of cells become insulin resistant our pancreas has to produce more insulin to be able to forcefully cram this extra sugar into our cells. Are we wearing out our pancreas by the type of foods we eat?

Low blood sugar is oft times caused by excess sugar: strange as it may sound, low blood sugar is often caused by excessive sugar and starch intake. When we take in foods that cause our blood sugar to spike, our pancreas has to produce a lot of insulin to bring the sugar down to safe levels. Insulin is a sugar hungry hormone that lowers blood sugar, so when there is an excessive spike in insulin, it causes our blood sugar to drop much lower than it should. Keep in mind that excess insulin also turns off the body's fat burning mechanisms.

This is a winnable war that we can win with a simple 2-prong strategy.

1. Increasing activity levels.

2. Having 4-5 grams of fiber per serving in our foods (except for some of the foods that we get our protein and fat from).

Given the role that excess sugar plays in diabetes, LDL cholesterol, obesity and all the potential side effects that can accumulate throughout a lifetime of controlling blood sugar with drugs), we have plenty of reason to want do this the right way!

Foods that are great for healing the pancreas: mushrooms, cherries, garlic, turmeric, tofu, yogurt, red grapes and spinach. Keep in mind that eating foods that break down slower also can be a big relief to the pancreas and in this way can have a healing effect as well.

Herbs, supplements etc. to control blood sugar: cinnamon, bitter melon, ginseng, chromium, bilberry, alpha-lipoic acid, fenugreek,

When we take the lazy way out by controlling our blood sugar for a lifetime of using a medication (so that we can continue to make the same food choices), we are simply setting ourselves up for failure.

When we control blood sugar spikes through food choices, activity and exercise, we also reduce excess fatty deposits and cholesterol!

Childhood Cancer and Our Early Donor Opportunity

 September is Childhood Cancer Awareness Month and brings attention to the trauma these children and their families go through that have to experience this. To see a child (and their family) going through this hurts deep and I can only imagine what a parent must be going through when they cannot absorb this hurt, pain and trauma their child is going through.

 Even though I'm a skeptic of the many "March Against This, March Against That events," there are some things I like in the awareness it brings to the prevention side for the real seekers and the ones who try to understand cancer and look beyond the barbaric treatment of cancer that cancer profiteers provide. The reason I consider these barbaric ways of treating cancer is surgery and biopsies seem to add fuel to the fire, the other two (chemotherapy and radiation) can damage the DNA of our cells and cells with damaged DNA reproduce warped versions of themselves which can lead to cancer.

We never know when these dreaded illnesses might visit our home, but there are things that we can do as a mother and father to build our baby's defenses against illness and disease prior to conception, during the pregnancy and the early years of our child's life.

Prior and during pregnancy: we have the opportunity as parents to build healthy gene expression throughout the beginning stages of our child's life from conception to birth. When we keep, toxic household chemicals, unhealthy diet, X-rays, CT scans, and other forms of radiation out of and away from our body prior to and during our pregnancy, we decrease our child's future risk of having cells produced the wrong way (aka cancer). During the pregnancy our child's immune system learns the things that should become accepted by their body after their birth by the things we subject them to while they are in the womb. After birth the things their body was not subjected to become anti-body and their immune system will attack it as a foreign invader! It's the things their body is too slow to recognize as foreign that we have to worry about. Our child's immune system is so powerful it can kill the entire body (such as in anaphylactic shock), so it can pretty much kill anything that it doesn't recognize as a part of our child's internal and external environment!

After birth: we have the opportunity during the years after our child's birth to build anti-cancer cells with nutrition, sunshine, exercise, regular rest and sleep habits that help fuel the growth of the next healthy generation of cells. As this process continues to grow, so does their capability snip out bad parts of DNA code that could build miss-shaped, misbehaving cells that could grow into cancer. This process helps nip the beginnings of cancer in the bud.

Living dirty and eating clean: two of the best ways I know to build the immune system is exposure and nutrition, the immune system also happens to be the thing that does battle against cancer in our child's body it only has to recognize these cells as foreign. Getting out in the sun, getting dirty, playing with siblings and friends, good diet along with consistent sleep and rest habits is a childhood cancer prevention lifestyle!

Household chemicals: most household chemicals are toxic (carcinogenic) and carcinogens cause cancer. Even though these cleaners may have the house smelling clean, we're turning it into a carcinogen trap and when we keep our children in an environment that is constantly being sanitized with toxic chemicals we increase theirs and our own susceptibility to cancer. There are safe household cleaners available, but if you're unsure of the carcinogenic effect of your cleaners, open windows and doors to air out your home (especially while cleaning), this helps lessen the toxic exposure.

Cancer is a devastating thing that can happen to anyone, but we as parents have a responsibility to do what we can to help our child build an immune system that works as a cancer shield in a cancerous world. Working our way backwards and learning what causes cancer (and turning off the faucet), is much more important then finding a cure...

 We as parents are builders of the home our child's life resides in. This building process starts before conception, goes through the early stages of childhood and impacts their habits and decisions as a young adult and helps set the foundation for the next generation. This is their body, they are our living legacy!

Your Child, Your Living Legacy

One of the best legacies we can leave here on earth is a son or daughter, and teaching them (the basics of health and nutrition can build their defenses in a world filled with bacteria's, germs, toxins, radiation and stress), is one of the best things we as parents can do for them.

September is Childhood Cancer Awareness month and instead of invoking fear in us, (to do a barrage of diagnostics, fundraising for the cure etc.) we should calm down and simply concentrate on implementing healthy habits in our children's lives that will strengthen their armor and help protect them from cancer and other diseases throughout their lives naturally.

Cancer is the second leading cause of death and as the medical community advances on heart disease (the number one cause of death) it may wind up becoming the leading cause of death for younger generations, if we do not change our approach and embrace the basic health principles that their bodies recognize as the cure. The 3 main strategies implemented by the cancer industry to date are pretty barbaric in their approach.

Cancer is a genetical disease (meaning it happens in the genes). This doesn't mean that it is inherited, but rather that it happens in the DNA of our cells. When we expose our cells to environmental toxins, food toxins, radiation and chemotherapy, and if our body cannot properly cleanse itself of these carcinogens and free radicals, it can have a corroding effect on the DNA of our cells. And since cells reproduce more cells the cells with corroded or corrupted DNA can produce weird shaped and misbehaving cells that we later recognized as cancer.

Example: a kitchen for a busy restaurant produces a massive amount of food. The recipes for this food come from a cookbook with many other recipes, (each one with its own special instructions for making the food). When the cook follows the exact recipe and process, the food will turn out the same every time a new batch of food is made, but what happens if he gets careless with the treatment of the cookbook, and the recipes get smeared and he is unable to properly transcribe (translate) the recipe for the new batches of food? The new batches of food can have a really funky turnout. Our children's cells are made in much the same way and when the recipe for the next generation of cells is not clear, it can produce weird shaped cells that (if not stopped by the body) can develop into an odd shaped lump that we later diagnose as cancer.

If a cell's DNA is messed up beyond repair there are mechanisms in place that cause these cells to commit suicide. After the cells die they become a waste product that the body can get rid of, this literally means that our body can clean up and dispose of cancer as we go.

Our responsibility as parents should be to put a protective screen around our children by the lifestyle we show and teach them. One of the best insurance policies that we can leave with them, are the good habits that have shaped who they are and who they will become.

Anti Cancer War Chest for children:

1. Fresh clean air.

2. Water.

3. Balanced diet with plenty of fruits and vegetables

4. Lots of physical activity and exercise.

5. Sunshine.

6. Deep rest.

7. Positive environment.

8. Consistency.

 May God bless your legacy with a lifetime of health!

Pathways To Suicide

This is a really hard subject, but one that most of us have already been affected by or will be in the future. I was at a visitation earlier this week for a friend of mine that gave up on life and a little while before I left for his visitation, a friend posted about a co-worker and friend that took her life. Just a little over a year ago my neighbor's young son took his life and within the same week one of my youngest members here at the gym took his life.

This is a really tough thing for family and close friends to go through, and leaves them with a constant stream of thoughts of what they could've said or done differently to change this final decision that was made.

I believe the reason more of a dialog isn't had between the public and the ones that study this, is due to what a lot of these cases trace back to and have in common with each other.

Example: there are many people that suffer from pain, depression and life altering tragedies, but what are the most common links that may factor in on the ones that choose to end it? Were they in intense pain? Were they in a deep depression? Did they go through a life-altering situation? Were they fixing the problem or were they medicating the problem? Was hope lost?

It can be easy to let the sadness and hurt turn to anger by the ones left behind as well as ones a little further removed from the situation to verbally or mentally judge a person or situation, but it is important to realize that we cannot properly judge a person who's shoes we have not personally walked in. And unless we know what it feels like to sink into a black hole of despair (without a glimmer or a ray of hope that things will get better), it is hard for us to understand.

Suicide from sudden impulse: I follow the research of a neurosurgeon (Dr. Russell Blaylock) and one particular article stood out to me where he spoke about the development (or underdevelopment) of the shadow region of the brain. He noticed how that attention spans were getting shorter when he gave class lectures, and he attributed this to rapid sources of information from tech devices. Accepting information at face value without research tends to not involve counter intuitive parts of the brain (shadow region) and when this is underdeveloped our capability to counter sudden thoughts with logic become less and less.

Example: if you have the sudden urge to hit someone that made you angry, what stopped you? Was it because they did something to calm you down or was it because you countered your anger with a host of reasons that you should not do this? When this part of the brain is not functioning or is not properly developed, a person's capability to counter sudden impulse is weakened.

 Pain and (or) disease: most times when we get hurt, have a chronic illness, debilitating condition or disease, and we have hope of getting rid of the pain or disease, it encourages us to fight our way back. But if it's a terminal disease, debilitating or deteriorating condition and if we are given no hope that the pain we are in will ever get better, a person may begin to look at their life as already being over and decide to end it. I personally believe the power for healing and recovery that is given to a person by his or her Creator should never be taken away by another human being.

The Mayo Clinic on pain and depression: pain and depression are closely related. Depression can cause pain and pain can cause depression. Sometimes pain and depression create a vicious cycle in which pain worsens symptoms of depression, and then the resulting depression worsens feelings of pain.

Suicide because of depression: depression can turn the lights of hope off in a person's brain and if not properly remedied can put a person in a very dark place. It may temporarily change someone's outlook by taking antidepressants, but it does nothing to change the depressing situation, just like pain pills do not remedy the pain your body is in, it simply makes so you can't feel it. I do not have answers for this since everyone's pain and depression is unique to them as an individual, but we should all realize that when we do not acknowledge pain and depression and do something real about what is causing it (instead of just medicating it), it tends to get worse.

Questions we should ask are: what is causing my body to hurt and what can I do to stop it? What is causing my depression and what can I do to make this situation better? What can I do to measure my actions so that I do not act on impulse in situations that may hurt myself or someone else?

There are pathways to suicide that can become highways for someone that loses hope. We can only try to create pathways for change and hope around ourselves and the ones we care about.

If you are someone that is contemplating this, just don't do it, you still have a purpose in making the lives better for the ones you care about, in the ways only you can.

If you lost someone you care about to suicide my prayer is that you will be able to find the happiness and peace that the one you are missing would want for you.

Are You At Risk For Breast Cancer?

Of course you are, if you have breast tissue (that is made up of glands, lobes, lobules, lymph vessels, lymph nodes etc.) then you are predisposed to cells potentially getting misshaped and then multiplying if not stopped. It's really nothing to get overly concerned about, since our body is constantly fixing things that are getting out of whack without us even knowing it. Each area of our body comes with its own system of cleansing, detoxification and repair mechanisms, so we should be looking for ways to strengthen that instead of constantly checking these areas to see if something is wrong with them.

Pre-cancer cells are a lot like someone being predisposed to potentially having a wreck because of being on the highway, but we're not going to spend a lot of time worrying about it or not driving our vehicle because of it are we? A wreck can be because of us not driving our vehicle carefully or it can be because of things out of our own control such as another driver, weather, etc. Either way, highway statistics should primarily encourage us to drive our vehicles safely, and to make sure we use standard preventive measures (that help our vehicle operate better) such as proper maintenance of breaks, tires, etc. We should not be constantly subjecting our vehicles to checkups by mechanics; especially ones that we do not personally know or we just may have a mechanic created vehicle problem.

We should not let ourselves be victimized by fear mongering when a doctor or oncologist tells us that we have pre-cancer cells, this is much like saying that due to the conditions of the highway you're traveling on your vehicle is pre-wreck. When you know the conditions on a highway are hazardous, you will try to take a different route and drive proactively and defensively to decrease your chances of having a wreck, right? Shouldn't our first priority be to change out any negative lifestyle habits for positive ones for our body as well? When we do this, our body can oft times create the right drugs and physiological processes (by itself) to shrink and annihilate cancer.

The month of October is breast cancer awareness month and is one of the biggest months of free advertising for the cancer industry, because of the fear and stress it creates. It probably causes more people to get unnecessary breast exams, mammograms and biopsies then any other time of the year. The ironic thing is mammography testing uses radiation and radiation damages DNA and damaged DNA is where most cancer begins.

"If you already have a cancer, in addition to being painful, the crushing compression the breast undergoes during a mammogram can cause the cancer to spread. Doctors are taught that once a lump is found, you don't press it, not even during an examination because you will cause the cancer cells to spread. With mammograms, you won't know if there is a breast cancer until after you've read the scan, you've already compressed the breast, and perhaps broken the cancerous capsule, which will cause the cancer to spread."

~ Dr. Russell Blaylock, Neurosurgeon and founder of the Blaylock Reports

If we would spend more time trying to figure out how to make our body parts feel good and healthy instead of trying to find out what might be wrong with them with diagnostics, prodding, biopsies and then the ensuing cancer treatments (that have been proven to cause other forms of cancer themselves later down the road), we would probably have much less new cancer cases, and an improvement in other aspects of health as well.

The cancer industry knows what causes cancer, and probably knows a lot about the dietary and lifestyle habits that will shrink and kill cancer, but the problem lies in that they cannot put a patent on nature or healthy lifestyle habits. One thing you can rest assured of is that for the ones at the top of most of these fundraisers and activities, it's not about finding a cure for cancer but much rather a way to find a breakthrough medication to manage it over the newly attained customer's lifetime. And yes, they do raise awareness, but isn't that how a business gains new customers? And yes, large portions of these fundraisers go to fund pharmaceutical research for creating new drugs. When pharmaceutical companies already make billions of dollars, why don't they fund their own research in creating for profit drugs?

Lets put at least 75% of our cancer awareness energy into finding a minimum of 10 dietary and lifestyle habits that will make our joints, tendons, ligaments, skin, muscles, digestive track, lymphatic system, brain, and other vital organs and systems feel better. And in the case of breast cancer, we should look for ways that we can make them feel better in such things as the environment they're continually exposed to as well as a good blood supply and lymphatic flow through the breast area.

Looking for a cure while ignoring the causes is like continually looking for ways to dry a floor while ignoring the leak and refusing to turn off the spigot.

After all it is the things that hurt our body parts in a continuous aggravating way that cause cancer.

Breast Environment

Our health is like a plant, our daily habits and environment is its soil...

One of the first things we should change when we have a body part or parts that are in pain (or if we want to prevent future pain or disease) is the lifestyle habits they're planted in. It is through our habits that both the good and bad things happening in our body get fed, (this shouldn't scare us, this should excite us)!

Example of good treatment: if we have a plant that is in a shaded area that doesn't get much sun, the dirt isn't very good, and we forget to water it, just imagine what would happen if we planted it in nutrient rich soil out front where it gets plenty of sunshine and plenty of attention. We would see this plant shed the old withered diseased leaves and begin to grow new ones, reflective of the simple changes in treatment it is getting.

Example of bad treatment: if we leave the same plant where it was and simply snip off, burn off, or use chemicals to get rid of the affected leaves and continue to forget to give it water and nutrients on a daily basis, wouldn't we be ignoring what is actually causing the problem in the first place?

One of the greatest contributors to cancerous mutations is ionizing radiation, and other forms of aggravation to a body part or organ, yet we radiate, press, probe, biopsy, cut and poison these areas of the body as a solution to a body part that is already hurting. Shouldn't we first try changing the environment and the soil we are planted in to see if this might shrink the problem into a non-issue?

What causes good breast cells to go bad: most of the cells of our body divide rapidly and this is no exception for breast tissue especially throughout the younger years. When the instructions for the new generation of cells gets corrupted and the built in mechanisms of the breast cells do not correct this, it can grow into something we later diagnosis as cancer. Radiation and carcinogens from our environment, food, etc., can change the structure of the DNA in our cells and when these cells replicate, they build cells that are not in synch with the others. If these corrupted breast cells break out of the area containing them (from compression or enzymatic breakdown of the wall) they can go to other areas of the body and grow corrupted breast tissue in that area.

The reason I do not believe in mammograms is that it exposes the breast tissue and heart area to ionizing radiation. Quite simply, it is using the very thing to detect cancer that also happens to cause cancer. The painful compressions of the breast tissue come before the mammogram and since doctors are taught to NOT compress after a lump is found (because it can break the cancerous capsule), is not this a direct contradiction of proper procedure?

Question: if oncology is going for early and safe detection, why is thermography not pushed more?

Thermography can detect unusual activity much earlier in the breasts then mammography and uses infrared imaging (which is safe) and does not use ionizing radiation.

"Our medical care system is rewarding doctors much more for ordering and reading scans than for talking to a patient." - "Radiation exposure from these scans is not inconsequential and can lead to later cancers." ~ Dr. Len Lichtenfeld Deputy chief medical officer for the national office of the American Cancer Society.

Allen Levin MD UCSF~ "Most cancer patients in this country die of chemotherapy. Chemotherapy does not eliminate breast, colon, or lung cancers. This fact has been documented for over a decade, yet doctor still use chemotherapy for these tumors."

Personal hypothesis: I believe we should be very careful what types of skin care products and deodorants we use regularly around the breast area and under our arms. I believe we should be careful what detergents we use on clothing and bed sheets that come in contact with our skin. I believe we should replace processed food and drinks with unprocessed foods. I believe many of the additives, chemicals and drugs we subject ourselves to can be hormone disrupters that become drivers of breast and other cancers. I believe we should stimulate breast tissue not mash, radiate and agitate it, (aggravation yields inflammation, continuous inflammation yields chronic inflammation and chronic inflammation yields cancer).

 I believe when we change the above and adapt healthy lifestyle habits that make our body feel better, we change the soil our health is planted in and our body parts will reflect our efforts.

Breast Cancer and Hormone Balance

Hormones are a signaling and messaging system that various cells, parts and systems of our body use to communicate with each other. If this gets out of whack it can cause things to operate differently, like a vehicle that needs to go forward but has been shifted in reverse.

When there is imbalance in estrogen production and a combination of cell injury in the breast area (from things such as excessive pressure, radiation, inflammation in the lymph nodes etc.), we are essentially priming this area for unusual cell growth.

Estrogen stimulates the growth of breast cell division and (since this is the primary breast hormone), if a breast cancer cell gets out of the original membrane pocket in the breast), these structurally messed up breast cells are drawn to other estrogen rich areas such as the ovaries and then can attach and grow there as well. When this happens, our immune system has a little extra work cut out for it. However if our immune system is strong, the only thing left for it to do is find the cancer, and a change in the diet can oft times make this much easier.

The EPA has an Endocrine Disrupter Screening Program (EDSP) and in 2012 released a list of 10,000 chemicals, (this document is 176 pages of chemicals and there are actually around 85,000 chemicals on the market). How can they keep up with the effects of these chemicals, (especially when used in combination with others), and how can we keep up with what these chemicals do to the chemistry of our body?

I believe we can over-stress about these things and that we should put our energy into things that strengthen our body's own defense. When we instead focus on how we can create a stable internal environment, (through our lifestyle habits) our body can deflect a lot of things around us that cause hormones to get out of balance, it then can create a homeostatic environment where hormones are balanced and metabolized properly. This is much better then excessive worry about factors we cannot control, our primary focus should be on the things we can.

Lifestyle factors that can affect estrogen levels: obesity, inactivity, alcohol, birth control pills, and hormone replacement therapy.

Here are some things that may help in winning the hormone-balancing act;

Frankincense: helps regulate production of estrogen- rub into breast area several times a week.

Cruciferous vegetables, such as broccoli, Brussels sprouts and cabbage, (can help the body excrete estrogen and other hormones). Regular consumption has shown powerful anti-breast cancer benefits. A Chinese study (Int J Cancer 2009;125:181-188) showed that one serving of cruciferous vegetables a day reduced the risk of breast cancer by 50%. A great way to release more of the hormone regulating, cancer fighting ICT's (isothiocyanate's) is to raw juice cruciferous vegetables. The list of anti-cancer benefits of cruciferous vegetables is an extensive one.

Turmeric (curcumin) has a potent phytoestrogen that can bind to estrogen receptors. Turmeric is also known for its powerful anti-inflammatory effects and since inflammation is at the root of cancer and the area of concern (breast cells) has estrogen receptors, it makes a whole lot of sense to me that turmeric (curcumin) is part of a daily supplement schedule.

Flaxseed is probably one of the highest add-ins that we can use in dietary lignan (a phytoestrogen compound). Phyto means from a plant and this being a plant estrogen should provide much the same benefits in blocking estrogen receptors.

Other sources of phytoestrogens are; sesame seeds, sunflower seeds, cashews, peanuts and poppy seeds.

Note: I believe there is more research that needs to be done on the effectiveness of phytoestrogens (in blocking estrogen receptors), but it makes sense that when an estrogen receptor is filled with a plant compound (phytoestrogen) it then can block it from receiving an estrogen. If the extra estrogen were floating around unable to attach itself to a receptor, wouldn't our body recognize it as waste it needs to metabolize and then clear it through our waste removal system?

Lifestyle habits to balance hormones:

1. Fresh clean air

2. Healthy balanced diet (using whole food).

3. Plenty of water (occasionally add electrolytes).

4. Exercise.

5. Sunshine (if you feel you're not getting enough, add vitamin D).

6. Deep sleep (with no stimulants or sugar 6 hours prior to bed time).

7. Last but not least, de-stress your life (this includes discounting advice from a doctor or oncologist that tries to push your panic buttons). It takes 7-10 years for a breast cancer to grow to a size that a mammogram can even detect, so you should never think that you have to do something NOW!

I believe very strongly in the power of the immune system and the lymphatic system's capability to govern the health of our body's systems and its parts, so one thing I believe would be of benefit to add in with the above is; a regular Manual Lymphatic Drainage Massage (apply less then 9 ounces of pressure per square inch and massage in a circular motion).

Hormones are messengers, and healthy lifestyle habits are what helps keep them balanced and from delivering weird messages to our corresponding, body parts or cells.

Breast Cancer Cell Apoptosis
"Nature's Chemotherapy"

In a study of over 10,000 patients, those who underwent chemotherapy were 14 times more likely to develop leukemia and 6 times more likely to develop cancers of the bones, joints, and soft tissue than those who did not undergo chemotherapy. (NCI Journal 87:10) John Diamond, MD.

Breast Cancer Awareness Month history: drug giant AstraZeneca (formerly Zeneca Group PLC) launched Breast Cancer Awareness Month in 1985. It wasn't started just to raise awareness but also to get more people talking about breast cancer as part of a national dialogue. This dialogue has served as a catalyst for generating a lot of fear in women about the possibility of developing breast cancer, which is probably a big reason that so many were convinced to get regular mammograms. Everything that I have researched about mammograms points toward usage of a technology (ionizing radiation) that is known to cause cancer and heavy compressions (which could possibly burst a pocket of cancer that we would be otherwise shielded from). So how does a drug company like AstraZeneca benefit from starting a movement such as Breast Cancer Awareness Month and partnering with many of the nation's leading cancer groups, such as American Cancer Society, and Susan G. Komen for the Cure to push for more cancer screenings? The answer may be found in knowing what 2 of their patented breast cancer blockbuster drugs are, Arimidex and Tamoxifen. These drugs are what tens of thousands of women are given after being diagnosed with breast cancer. So were they the wolf the FDA has been letting guard our henhouse?

Ionizing radiation of the breasts (mammograms) has been pushed for many years for both the young, middle age and elderly, now suddenly it appears that an attempt at a soft back down is happening by the same organizations that pushed massive usage of this cancer causing form of diagnostics. They are now recommending using it at an older age but are still not mentioning thermography, (a diagnostic technology that can detect unusual breast cell activity long before mammography does without doing any harm to breast tissue).

We have seen time and again that surgery oft times seems to be like giving oxygen to a fire, we know that chemotherapy is a carcinogen (carcinogens cause cancer) and ionizing radiation causes cancer, so why do we do these things to help us win the cancer battle? Beats me! I spoke to one of my members today that recently had a biopsy done on a growing spot on one of his lungs, there were 6 chunks taken out of this area and his lung collapsed. Even though they were able to find out what it is, isn't this a terribly invasive approach to an already hurting area of the body? What if we could strengthen the body and its discovery mechanisms, which in turn can cause cancer cell apoptosis (cell suicide) selectively to the cancer cells?

Apoptosis: there are lots of natural chemicals in our foods that cause corrupted (cancerous) cells to die. These natural foods also help regular cells become stronger and healthier. When we strengthen from within the stem cells, the cells they produce become stronger and better regulated. As the surrounding cells get healthier and stronger, so does the body's capability to dispose of the cancerous cells and new healthy tissue can grow there instead!

I've been trying to uncover the best foods, seeds etc. for boosting the body's natural capability of apoptosis of cancer cells and this is what I found;

Fruits: wild blackberry, strawberry, choke cherry, elderberry, avocado, black raspberry, jamun berry (Indian blackberry).

Seeds: apricot seed, peach seed, apple seed, cherry seed, nectarine seed, pear seed, plum seed, prune seed. These seem to be some of the biggest cancer fighters.

Nuts: bitter almond, macadamia.

Leaves: alfalfa, eucalyptus.

Herbs: marijuana (especially the tetrahydrocannabinol or THC).

Teas: Essiac tea, green tea, pine. One that is of special interest since I live in the south is the steeping of pine needles into a tea.

Roots: garlic and ginger. Ginger has been shown to selectively kill breast cancer cells. **PMID: 22969274**

Miscellaneous: baking soda, turmeric, vitamin D, dark chocolate, and kale.

 We tend to avoid bitter tasting foods, seeds, grasses, teas etc. but I believe this is a good indicator of its effectiveness and medicinal capabilities. I also believe we should go primarily for foods, herbs, teas, spices etc. that are grown in our home area.

 One of the best ways to put on a protective breast guard that will help protect against breast cancer is healthy, consistent lifestyle habits. Doing this, not only can protect us from cancer, it can also shrink and eliminate the cancer. When we adapt healthy habits, our immune system and health can start immediately improving instead of getting slammed as most conventional (for profit) cancer treatment protocols do!

Chemotherapy, radiation and surgery have been major detractors not so much in actually shrinking the cancer problem, but rather in an increase in reliance on things that oft times seem to exasperate a problem and further wound an already hurting body. We have many things around us that nature provides that bring both balance and healing. But once again, these things are not patentable so the funds raised by Susan G. Komen for the Cure, American Cancer Society and others are not going into studying the medicine that nature provides, but rather promoting the business of screenings, patentable medicines laboratories provide.

Holding Your Breath

A common expression is don't hold your breath especially when it comes to things that are not going to happen. This term is used a lot in the gym as well, but is there times when holding or slightly holding our breath can be a good thing? Can this help brace us or strengthen us internally for handling external forces?

Quite often when a person has chronic joint pain, they can feel pressure changes from the weather and some can even tell if it's going to rain. When there is enough of a pressure difference in our external environment vs. our internal pressure it can be felt by pain in joints, especially if there is inflammation in these areas. So if we can figure out how to counter the pressure from the outside with that of the inside, maybe we can have a skeletal structure that is less affected by outside forces.

Protecting our back: when we breathe in deeply and slightly hold our breath during the primary exertion phase of lifting something, the air we are holding works from the inside a lot like a support belt does from the outside in supporting our spine.

Example: imagine lifting something very heavy and setting it on a top shelf. Then imagine doing this with all your air exhaled out, it would make your back feel like it's going to cave in. At least partially holding your breath during a lift like this can really help internally stabilize your back. Smoothly exhale as you're completing the lift.

How holding your breath can make you stronger: the Vasalva maneuver is something most of us use fairly regularly at varying intensities without even thinking about what we're doing or even knowing what the Vasalva maneuver is.

Method: the Vasalva maneuver is done by taking in a breath of air and then pushing the air up against a closed airway. In this case the closed airway is the glottis (the opening between the vocal cords). This pressure inside the chest area forces blood out of the pulmonary circulation and into the left atrium of the heart (which is where our oxygenated blood goes before being sent out to the rest of the body). This often gives us a surge of power for a short duration.

Vasalva maneuver for inner ear pressure: we can use the Vasalva maneuver as well when going through the mountains, valleys or air travel when we feel pressure building up in our head.

Method: breathe in deep, close your mouth, hold your nose shut and then slowly push the air up from your lungs (like you're going to force it out of your nose). You will usually feel air push through the Eustachian tube of the middle ear, like a pressure release valve.

Blood pressure warning: overuse of the Vasalva maneuver (against the glottis) can cause potential high spikes of blood pressure due to the air pressure around the upper heart and lung area. Exhaling slowly during the lift can help keep blood pressure from spiking and the subsequent drop in pressure when blood returns to normal circulation. I do not recommend the Vasalva maneuver for more then 3-5 seconds at a time and if it's multiple repetitions, I would highly recommend a steady flow of breathing. The above is not something we have to overly concern ourselves with since most of the time proper breathing comes naturally without us needing to pay extra attention to it.

 When we inhale and get extra oxygen along with a slight increase in blood pressure we become more alert, energized and stronger, when we exhale, we tend to become more relaxed.

 Proper breathing technique: inhale as you lower the weight and exhale slowly as you lift the weight, likewise if it's a pulling exercise, inhale as you pull, exhale as you release. Using proper breathing technique should give you an increase in strength and support your back!

Imagine it like this: during the easy part of the movement breathe in a full breath of air and as you go through the exertion part of the movement (such as pushing the bar up from the chest while bench pressing), slowly release your breath. Likewise in a squatting movement, breathe in as you're going into the squat position and exhale as you're going back into the standing position. This should give you give you the maximum benefit of spinal support and extra strength without the spike in blood pressure.

 We use this process without thinking most times, especially when we're bracing ourselves for a heavy load. Even a baby does it naturally when they are clenching their little fists and getting red in the face when they're trying to get rid of a load!

 I'm not sure exactly what physiological effect that happens to cause the body to temporarily strengthen when we do this, but I do think it's pretty awesome that the same thing that gives us a temporary surge in strength, also protects our back!

Is Your Muscle In A Pickle?
Try Pickle Juice...

Just recently after a hard leg workout I got a very uncomfortable round of leg cramps. Most times I'm moving around a good bit after a workout, but this time I was mostly sitting at the desk or on the road, so my legs had the opportunity to stiffen up. Out of curiosity I started researching the cause or physiology of cramps.

This is the best explanation I found: cramps can occur when muscles are unable to relax properly due to myosin fibers not fully detaching from actin filaments. In skeletal muscle, adenosine triphosphate (ATP) must attach to the myosin heads for them to disassociate from the actin and allow relaxation, the absence of ATP in sufficient quantities means that the myosin heads remain attached to actin.

What this means to me: when muscle energy (ATP) is low it can cause the muscle to get stuck in a contracted position instead of the normal sliding back and forth. So if ATP depletion happens when we work our muscles more then they're used to getting worked, it stands to reason that our muscle glycogen (muscle energy) that is used for ATP, is low in this overworked area and we have a fuel shortage. At this point a quick absorbing fluid with carbohydrate/sugar/glucose may help.

A really neat function of the body is its ability to direct nutrients to the highest demand areas first. One of the best things we can do to enhance transport of these nutrients is physical movement and I have noticed when I do an active cool down and light stretching after a workout, I don't have cramps. Could this mean that when we deplete the energy in a muscle group, the physiology of light movement (of these areas) helps pump in hydration and nutrients to build new ATP in these areas that just caught the shaft?

Note: if you have problems cramping during physical activity, try warming up this area of the body with light activity about 5 minutes prior to the intense activity. This should increase blood flow and nutrients into this area and work in much the same way as light activity and stretching after intense activity.

One of my elderly members was having problems with cramps and when I asked about her diet, I found out that she makes most of her food and pretty much had salt eliminated from her diet. After suggesting adding in extra salt her problems with cramping seemed to go away. However most of us probably get more then enough salt if we eat restaurant prepared foods regularly. I would aim for about 3/4 - 1-teaspoon daily depending on activity levels and bodyweight. This would come to approximately 1,725 - 2,300 mg of sodium. Our daily amount doesn't have to stay the same, if we take in more or less then we should one day, we can simply adjust our intake the next day. However if you have blood pressure or water retention problems I would keep the amount per meal monitored closely.

Pickle juice: my cramping disappeared soon after drinking about 2-3 oz. of pickle juice and eating one, so I decided to look at the ingredients in a jar of pickle juice and work my way backwards to learn a little more about the individual ingredients that make up pickles and their juice. I wanted to see what makes it so effective and to possibly get a better picture of what causes a cramp in the first place.

The most obvious ingredients are: cucumbers, water, vinegar, sea salt, calcium chloride and sodium benzoate.

Cucumbers: cucumbers are primarily made up of water and help us hydrate. They also contain potassium and potassium helps maintain good muscle contraction all over the body and helps ensure that our central nervous system works well. Without getting a lab analysis done, I'm not sure how this applies to the juice but I have used pickle juice only and it works the same way in relieving cramps.

Vinegar: vinegar is known not only for its food flavoring and pickling capabilities but also for powerful medicinal effects dating back to Hippocrates. And if it permeates our muscle cells like its flavor permeates food it may be a good reason it also gets to the cramp site as rapidly as it does.

Sea salt: Our body is 75% water and the water that is held in our cells, tissues and organs is a salty watery solution similar to that of the ocean. Sea salt has other minerals in it as well so sea salt is definitely my preference.

Calcium chloride: increases cell membrane permeability.

Sodium benzoate: helps liberate heat and is used as a treatment for urea cycle disorders due to its ability to bind to amino acids. This leads to excretion of these amino acids and a decrease in ammonia levels.

I'm sure each of the ingredients listed above have many other usages or applications, but I only zeroed in on the ones that seemed might apply to cramp relief.

Question: if ATP (muscle energy) is lacking and causing muscle fibers to stick together and if pickle juice helps remedy this, is it possible that consuming a little pickle juice before extreme exertion, long bouts of activity or a workout might increase muscle energy and help prevent cramps as well?

Either way, it seems pickle juice might have more value then just keeping the dills wet until consumption!

Pancreatic Cancer and Diabetes

November is awareness month for both pancreatic cancer and diabetes. I doubt this is coincidental since both have to do with the pancreas. Our pancreas produces enzymes for digestion and is our source for insulin, which helps transport glucose from our blood into the cells of our body.

If we link diabetes and pancreatic cancer together and look at both as a result stemming from repeat injury to the pancreas, I believe it will give us better insight as to the root causes of either.

Pancreatic cancer is one of the most fatal forms of cancer and diabetes is an issue that many of us are facing now or will in our future if we do not make changes. However if we make lifestyle changes that heal the pancreas we may be able to not only side step the progression of either of these diagnosis's, we just might be able to shrink either one into insignificance even after diagnosis.

Pancreatic cancer: if we look at the precursor of cancer, (chronic inflammation) and look for what is causing the inflammation (pancreatitis) in the pancreas, we should be able to trace the origin of the problem. When we lighten the load on the pancreas by eating less processed sugars, less meat and more whole unprocessed food, not only should pancreatic performance get better, it should help heal a hurting pancreas as well. According to the American Cancer Society pancreatic cancer is more common in people who have diabetes, so it seems pretty obvious that they may stem from some of the same sources of continued aggravation, which will initially yield the medical diagnosis of pancreatitis, which is simply inflammation of the pancreas. If this smoldering inflammation (chronic pancreatitis) continues, it can become cancer.

The most common causes of pancreatitis are gallstones and heavy alcohol use. It's not hard to figure out how to cut out the aggravation from alcohol, (we can simply eliminate our intake).

However gallstones (the most common cause) is the one that may be a little more complicated.

Gallstones: there is a theory that gallstones form because of bile containing too much cholesterol. Normally our bile contains enough chemicals to break down the cholesterol excreted by our liver, but if the liver excretes more cholesterol than our bile can dissolve, the excess cholesterol may form into crystals and eventually into stones. This makes sense because of the gallbladder holding this bile until we need it for fat digestion and if this bile has too much un-dissolved cholesterol in it, it makes sense as well that it could form little balls of hard cholesterol (gallstones) if stored too long.

Gallstone and pancreas connection: gallstones can block the shared bile duct which can block pancreatic enzymes from going into the small intestine and in turn forces them back up into the pancreas. The enzymes then begin to irritate the cells of the pancreas, causing the inflammation associated with pancreatitis. If we can get to the bottom of why these little boogers calcify and form maybe we can eliminate the primary aggravation that leads to pancreatitis and the possible root cause of pancreatic cancer and diabetes (or at least the form of diabetes where the pancreas is unable to produce an adequate amount of insulin). There is also a form of diabetes where your cells have so much insulin coming at them (from all the sugar intake) that they eventually become insulin resistant.

 The best ways to sidestep all the complicated medical and nutritional jargon above can be summed up through 2 words, DIET & EXERCISE!

 The next chapter will be on healing the pancreas and naturally flushing the gallbladder. If we can lighten the load on our pancreas, it just might help us avoid pancreatic cancer and diabetes. We can have small amounts of cancer in an organ such as the pancreas and never know it, but it can certainly affect its performance!

Flushing Gallstones and Healing Our Pancreas

Our pancreas does a massive amount of work in helping our body break down and absorb nutrients from our diet, so if we don't give back, it can become overworked and potentially diseased. When it becomes fatigued or diseased our chances of diabetes can increase as well as our capability to digest our foods decrease. There are a few steps we can take if we feel our pancreas is in trouble.

1. Gallbladder flush: our gallbladder was given to us for a reason and my personal opinion is that we should try a flush before we let the medical field surgically remove it because of stones. Though this is not endorsed by the medical field, this is what I would do to get rid of stones: very low fat diet for 5 days (this will increase your gallbladder's sensitivity to fat) and should increase the concentration of bile in the gallbladder, which may make the stones smaller during this 5 day period. Consume 2-3 apples a day, (the pectin in apples supposedly softens the stones). After the 5 days, (on the evening of the 5th day) skip dinner and around 6 pm mix 1 teaspoon of Epson salt (magnesium sulphate) in a glass of warm water and then again at 8 pm. These 2 rounds of Epson salt will help dilate and relax the gallbladder ducts. At 10 pm mix a 1/2 glass of olive oil with a 1/2 glass of lemon juice. Since your diet has been so restricted from fat, the gallbladder should be very sensitive to all the olive oil and should put out a lot of bile. Because the Epson salt has dilated and relaxed the gallbladder ducts, the stones should be able to drop out rather easily.

2. Gall stone prevention: clearing our gallbladder from stones helps ensure the shared duct (our pancreas uses to drip enzymes into our digestive tract as our food passes through) stays clear. Consuming lots of water, and a fiber rich diet with plenty of green leafy vegetables, legumes (kidney beans, black beans, soybeans), Atlantic cod, salmon, eggs, milk, peanuts and other foods high in lecithin may keep gallstones from forming, by keeping them in a dissolved state. Eat vitamin C rich foods, (you can also add a vitamin C supplement to your diet).

 The above listed foods can assist in turning the cholesterol into bile acid and if we can have a stronger bile acid mixture in our gallbladder (bile storage tank) we can possibly avoid this excess cholesterol from forming lumps (gallstones). It makes sense that if this bile becomes strong enough in our gallbladder it should dissolve stones as well. The addition of wheat bran, wheat germ, spinach and beets are a great food source for Betaine, which helps with bile flow.

3. Foods and herbs that heal the pancreas system:

Mushrooms are shown to help block the MMP gene that has been linked to the development of pancreatic cancer.

Cherries are a rich source of antioxidants and perillyl alcohol a compound proven to help prevent pancreatic cancer.

Garlic, onions, chives, fenugreek, shallots and leeks contain sulfur, arginine, selenium, oligosaccharides and flavonoids that have been shown to prevent pancreatic cancer.

Turmeric is shown to be effective against many cancers, including pancreatic cancer.

Yogurt and other probiotic rich foods help aid the digestive system and should provide some relief to the pancreas. Btw do not use the yogurt that tastes like sweetened pudding, (use the unsweetened kind). The medical experts at the German Institute of Human Nutrition Potsdam-Rehbrueke recommend the best way to protect your pancreas and lower risk of pancreatic cancer is to consume a diet high in spinach or more specifically leafy green veggies such as kale, spinach, mustard greens, and Swiss chard with elevated levels of B vitamins and iron.

If you've had your gallbladder removed, I would highly recommend regularly eating foods rich in choline (such as salmon, eggs, dark chocolate, beef liver etc.) and Betaine rich foods (such as wheat germ, wheat bran, beets and spinach). Betaine helps with the natural breakdown of fat; choline helps with the absorption of fat and cholesterol. Keep a bile salt supplement for times you slip up and consume a meal with too much fat or greasy food.

Our pancreas and gallbladder help with digestion and the breaking down of food particles into nutrients that our body can absorb. The health of especially the pancreas is vital for overall health of the body and is a big factor in helping us to sidestep diabetes, after all the pancreas is our body's natural insulin pump!

The next chapter will be on what we can do to prevent diabetes, and no longer live diabetic.

Reversing Diabetes

Don't ever underestimate the power of the body to reverse symptoms when the cause is taken away and healing lifestyle changes take its place!

Whenever a medical term is used with pre (in front of the diagnosis) and we are sold on the idea that it should be medicated instead of us making applicable changes to our lifestyle, we are succumbing to a proposed remedy that oft times does not have a good history of bearing good fruit compared to simply making these lifestyle changes.

Tracing type 2 diabetes back to where it originates from is as simple as **1-2-3.**

1. An over worked pancreas.

2. Cells of the body that have gotten insensitive to insulin.

3. Then we need to ask ourselves why our

pancreas is getting overworked and why our cells have gotten insensitive to insulin?

The answers to these questions will give us a solution to cure our problem, not just help us manage it.

 Over worked pancreas: our pancreas is responsible for a lot of digestive enzymes and the insulin our body uses to help move glucose from our blood to our cells. When we are eating sugar or "starch heavy meals" almost every time we eat, our pancreas has to work like crazy to keep up. When the cells of our body are constantly bombarded with insulin they gradually become insensitive to it (or become calloused to it). This forces the pancreas to produce even more insulin to force uptake of the sugars in our diet (this is a little like having to shout your message to a person that is going deaf because of all the racket his or her ears have to constantly endure). This forces your pancreas to work much harder then it should and creates insensitivity to insulin. If we can create a greater sensitivity to insulin we can remedy and provide relief to our overworked pancreas.

Steps we can take to sidestep and reverse diabetes:

1. One of the best ways to increase insulin sensitivity is to decrease the sugar in our diet, (in other words, if it tastes sweet don't eat or drink it). When everything goes quiet for long enough in a loud room, after a while our ears will be able to hear the slightest noise. It's much the same with our cells when we decrease the amount of circulating sugar, (over time they will become more sensitive to insulin). And when our pancreas doesn't have to produce as much, it can get some much-needed relief.

2. Insulin is a hormone and it simply tells the cells that there is glucose available and triggers mechanisms inside the cell that helps draw glucose inside. But if the cells cannot understand the message, they will not draw the glucose into the cell for nourishment and energy.

3. Intermittent fasting (IF) is one of my favorite ways to drop body fat and has also been shown to help slow the progression and even reverse diabetes. Fasting helps clear excess fat from our liver and if we can keep our energy laboratory in good lean condition, it should go a long ways toward helping us keep blood glucose levels steady.

Glut4: Our cells have something called GLUT4 (glucose transporter type 4) in them. Glut4 is our cell's way of inserting little suction straws out through the membrane of our cells so we can draw glucose into the cell (insulin triggers this). We can stimulate these Glut4 receptors to the surface of our cells with muscle contraction. So when we purposely make muscles work hard all over our body, our capability to absorb sugar into the muscle goes up and the need for excess insulin goes down. Increasing muscle contractions is to our muscle cells like wearing hearing aids (instead of earmuffs) is to our ears, it increases their capability to draw in and process glucose.

Blood glucose lowering tool chest:
cinnamon, ginger, ginseng, chromium, magnesium, vinegar, and ALA (Alpha-Lipoic Acid) are known to help lower blood glucose levels.

In a nutshell: we can tell by looking at the origin of the most prominent form of diabetes (type 2) that it comes from excess sugar intake and inactivity. If we do the opposite we can squash this epidemic.

When we remove the earmuffs from our cells and give them hearing aids instead, our pancreas does not have to speak so loudly (with the amount of insulin it has to produce) and we can bring restoration to a tired, irritated and inflamed pancreas while restoring health and energy to the cells of our body without a needle or a pill! In this way, we may be able to lower our risk for diabetes and pancreatic cancer!

H.I.V. And The Immune System

 As of the end of 2014 there were approximately 37 million people worldwide living with HIV (Human Immunodeficiency Virus). Most of us probably already know this disease compromises the immune system and (most anyone that knows me), knows my passion for the human body's immune system and how we can naturally stimulate it. My interest is not so much in HIV as it is in this virus's interest in the immune system. Why is this virus so attracted to the human body's T helper cells? What can we learn about the devastating effects of a continually compromised immune system that will show us what we can prevent with a strong immune system?

 The breakdown of HIV is this:

H: Human - a virus infecting humans.

I: Immunodeficiency - a weakening of the immune system's CD4 cells also known as T helper cells.

V: Virus - a virus can only reproduce itself by taking over a cell in the body; it is incomplete and ineffective until then.

The basics of HIV makes it a lot like other viruses in that it needs the components of a human cell to replicate itself. It's like a foreigner wanting to use a domestic factory (that has the machines they need) to build their poison products with the intention of destroying the country that the factory is in. The best way to keep this from happening is to prevent foreign invasion at all entry points and not letting someone use the factory equipment that shouldn't be.

The virus: the protein on this particular virus is particularly attracted to and almost seems like it was tailor designed to perfectly fit the receptors on one of our immune system's main components (T helper cells) and in turn use them as a factory to reproduce replicas of the virus.

The immune system and HIV: our immune system is our intelligence and defense system that recognizes what is foreign to the body and what is actually self. Since T cells are a large part of our immune system, (when the HIV virus infects them) it will gradually slow down this system's capability to detect foreign invaders. It is like a country (that is surrounded by other countries) that slowly over time gets rid of their intelligence and military personnel; it simply makes the country vulnerable to opportunistic countries that prey on another country's weakness. This weakness can lead to a country's demise.

This encroachment of the body's immune system cells can go for a long time (our immune system is powerful and can fight back), but if a person with HIV does not have a good counter punch strategy, their resistance to illness and disease can weaken much sooner.

AIDS (acquired immunodeficiency syndrome): is the final stage of HIV and is the point the person with HIV pretty much has lost his/her defenders and is vulnerable to most any opportunistic infectious invaders that prevail themselves as cancers, neurological problems or other illness. This is pretty much when the homeland is left completely unguarded and without protection against invaders from the outside.

Whether you have HIV, AIDS, or simply want to build a strong defense to stay healthy and strong, there are a few simple steps you can take.

Building and maintaining a strong immune system:

1. Detox: one of the first things is to free up your immune system to only work on new things (this can be done by cleaning up the colon and getting rid of old stuff our body is continuing to absorb and then have to detox itself from). I would recommend a 7 day guided system detox. A high fiber diet (with plenty of organic fruits and vegetables) will help detox the other digestive organs. You can add Psyllium husk fiber as well. Doing these things help keep the bowels scrubbed clean and helps drag toxins out of our wastebasket.

2. Build gut health: a large part of our immune

system is generated from our digestive tract. Raw fruits and vegetables, fermented product such sauerkraut and cultured cabbage juice as well as adding in probiotics help restore digestive health.

Study up as much as you can on gut health.

3. Healthy habits done with consistency: Good deep rest, activity, breath clean air, stay hydrated with water, sunshine and stay stress free along with a good social circle of family and friends.

I want to thank my uncle (Dr. Kauffman) for his help with this article. He specializes in HIV and has done a lot on the mission field for HIV and AIDS patients. Your immune system works like a medical team 24-7-365 days a year; it is your defense system.

Understanding The Baby Language Of Our Parts

Mathew 7:9~ Which of you, if your son ask for bread, will give him a stone instead?

 Most adults at one point or the other have been around a baby or babies that were crying and probably got pretty desperate trying to figure out what it is that they wanted or what was bothering them. And probably quite often had the uncomfortable feeling of giving something or doing the wrong thing and the baby getting even more upset.

 When we know our baby really well it can help prevent mistakes and help us have a much healthier happier child. After all why would we want to give our child medicine when it has an upset stomach because of the food he or she is eating? Why would we want to give them a pacifier when they are hungry or thirsty? Why would we want to give them pain medicine without first checking to make sure their environment is really comfortable for their tiny and tender bodies? And why would we give them a toy when what they really want is our attention?

Our body parts are much the same in what they want from us as well. They want us to figure out what they are trying to tell us, and are not wanting us to take a lazy shortcut to pacify them temporarily or worse yet take medicine that makes so we cannot feel their pain.

Most of our symptoms come from underlying pain that a body part or system is going through and when we take a medicine instead of making the appropriate lifestyle change(s) that our body part is asking for we are in turn asking for a fountain of medical health issues.

Example: if our knee is hurting really bad and we take pain medicine instead of putting on a knee wrap (to lighten the load), we are telling our knee to shut up and to just deal with whatever is hurting it. It's like putting a pair of earmuffs on and acting like your baby isn't crying, except it is still crying and since you are ignoring it, the problem is only going to get worse.

 When we can get tuned in with our body and its parts, being able to track what is hurting it will become easier. Though the easy path of medicine (that addresses symptoms but does not change what is causing the symptoms) may be an easy path temporarily, it does not lead in a good direction.

 "Ask why, and ask it again five more times, until all of the artifice is stripped away and you end up with the intellectually honest answer."

~ Andy Grove

 Listening to your body and what it is trying to tell you is important, after all if you do not listen to your body who else will? You are the parent of your body parts.

Freedom From Drugs vs. Cheap Access To Drugs

We live in an era where there is far too much emphasis on cheap or free access to drugs and healthcare and not enough emphasis on doing what we can to live drug-free and to be less reliant on the healthcare system instead of relying so heavily on it for our health and wellbeing. We oft times look at people that are on drugs illegally as being "on drugs" while we ourselves are putting our bodies and organs through hell on legal drugs. How much does our body actually care about what is legal or illegal?

Why is it that we think that a man-made pill from the opium plant is okay to use in mass quantities throughout the United States? The easy access to these narcotics and the low bar set for prescriptions should be clear as crystal to the regulators as to why there is such a problem with massive usage and distribution of these.

Note: Afghanistan is the primary producer of the world's opium. The Taliban decreased production in Afghanistan by 94% in 2000, but after the American and British invasion of Afghanistan in 2001, and the installation of the interim government, Afghanistan once again became the world's largest producer of opium. When you look at the massive consumption of pain pills (made from opioids) here in the United States it does not take a rocket scientist to figure that one out.

Our real addiction: we use drugs to manage symptoms instead of relieving our hurting body part(s) or system(s) of the actual problem. This applies to diabetes management, arthritis management, pain management, cholesterol management, blood pressure management, cancer management and the list goes on and on. When we take drugs for symptoms but are unwilling to change the lifestyle habit that is causing it, (though it is accepted in today's society and condoned by the FDA) our body's opinion is quite simply that; we are a drug user and abuser.

We have a new year coming up and one thing that we can all benefit from is decreasing our dependence on drugs whether illegal or legal (including alcohol and tobacco), and making the lifestyle changes that empower our body to make its own personal designer drugs it needs to fight the bad stuff and to keep us healthy. There are some things that we can do now to help prevent or decrease our dependence on drugs in 2016.

Statins: instead of using statin drugs to manage cholesterol, let's start making the dietary changes needed to heal our network of blood vessels (taking away the reason for the cholesterol sticking to our blood vessel walls), lower our sugar and high fructose corn syrup intake and increase fiber intake. Increasing our fiber intake causes us to lose bile that our body has to replace), our liver then makes new bile from cholesterol, which lowers our cholesterol. That's why high fiber foods are considered cholesterol-lowering foods.

Sugar lowering drugs and insulin: we can lower our need for insulin and sugar lowering drugs through diet and exercise. Exercise helps suck up glucose from the blood to energize our muscles thus lowering blood sugar. Intense exercise stimulates the hormone Glut4 to the surface of our muscle cells and helps sugar enter into them easier, lowering the amount of insulin we need. This helps lower the stress put on our pancreas for insulin production.

Blood pressure drugs: a heart healthy diet with healthy dietary fats and an active lifestyle can decrease our need for blood pressure medicine. A quick remedy for blood pressure is doing slow to moderate activity until you feel your body heat up. This causes blood to heat up as well (blood that is heated up relaxes blood vessels).

Drugs for gastro intestinal issues: keep a food diary for what you eat and how you feel. This timeline will give you a prescription of what you need to eliminate (that your gut doesn't like) and may also help you resolve autoimmune disorders that can be caused by un-dissolved food particles getting into your blood. Un-dissolved particles can cause our organs to get inflamed when the blood delivers food particles instead of nutrients that are ready to absorb.

Pain drugs: finding out why our body part or system is hurting and then eliminating this will dry out the inflammation that is causing the pain. When a pain gets too intense in an area, cool it down; this helps shrink the inflammation thus reducing the pain.

Even though we can find out many of the side effects of individual drugs, there is very little research if any on long-term effects of drug combinations.

Giving your body the chance to work its way through things by giving it time and good lifestyle habits can decrease your dependence on drugs produced by man and will build a stronger and more skilled immune system that can build the exact drugs your body needs.

Continued use of medications, (especially multiple ones) work in the body like an unlabeled mixed pack of seeds does in the ground; you really don't know what the results will yield. Let's make it our mission to find the reasons our body needs a drug in the first place and eliminate that which will take away the need for the drug or at the least help decrease the dosage and frequency.

"The best doctors give the least medicines."
~Benjamin Franklin

Heath and Fitness Notes

To attempt to live longer is Nuts!: research has shown that death from the leading causes of death (heart disease, cancer and respiratory), were lower in ones with a higher nut consumption. Use local grown nuts replace unhealthy snacks.

Fitness starting points: 1. Gain muscle. **2.** Lose body fat. **3.** Increase endurance. **4.** Fight disease by empowering your own immune system; it produces its own drugs when we do that.

Detox for prevention energy and fitness: keeping our body toxin free, helps us to not only unleash the power of the immune system, but happens to slenderize the waist as well! Oft times a good detox can get rid of 7-12 pounds of waste!

Too much exercise can clog up your drainpipes: over doing it can cause too much protein breakdown and overwhelm the kidneys. Steady wins the race!

You are Trillions: your body is made up of

trillions of cells, (most of which regenerates at least once a year). Your habits can rejuvenate or age your cells.

Hormone imbalance: keeping a good diet, plenty of water, active lifestyle, deep rest and getting rid of stress helps go a long ways in keeping our hormones balances.

This little pump inside our chest: our heart pumps around 20 quarts of blood per minute (at rest) and will pump a total of around 1.5 million gallons of blood (into a network of approximately 50,000 miles of blood vessels) every year for us!

The basics for heart health are: fresh clean air, heart healthy balanced diet, sunshine, staying hydrated with clean water, exercise, deep rest, sleep, stress release, fun, and quality time spent with the ones you care about!

Renewing our worn out joints: why is it that people who are told, they HAVE TO HAVE back or knee surgery, are immediately upon diagnosis prescribed pain pills, pain blocks, and anti-inflammation drugs instead of a back belt, decompression therapy, knee support, and joint building supplements (between diagnosis and time of surgery)? But then why would a salesman want to show you how you can avoid doing business with him?

What soil is your health and fitness planted in?: our health and fitness has roots, and it is planted squarely in the lifestyle habits we choose and oft times the environment we select. This defines the outcome much like nutrient rich soil and hydration does for a plant. Each choice we make determines the dirt our health and fitness is planted in.

Restoring old fat "cellulite": cellulite is blood and oxygen starved fat. We can help smooth and repair this fat by building a better blood flow to this area, building muscle in this area, and increase blood flow into these areas by applying heat and skin brushing.

Bottom to the top: too often we feel change uses a top down approach but I think its pretty clear to most of us by now, that change is not going to happen at the top unless the soil (that gives problems a root system to grow in) changes! Your purchases, your vote, your lifestyle is this soil and what grows on top represents you! Even though our action or inaction may seem like a little pebble dropped in a massive lake, the ripple effect can last a lifetime and longer! Sometimes change has to happen at the bottom, for change to happen at the top...

Functional training for real life function: exercising your muscles in the manner you use them in real life will strengthen and empower movement. This trains you like an athlete instead of a bodybuilder, ever notice how stiffly many bodybuilders move?

April...cancer control month?: when did the language change from "The search for a cure" to "Cancer Control?" The nearest cure we will probably ever find is prevention through lifestyle. It would be stupid for business if the cancer industry to come up with a cure, they like residual income too!

Homeostasis vs. Cancer: homeostasis is simply a state of normal that our body tries to return to no matter if we get dehydrated, cold, hot, sick, infections or even get emotionally upset. This list of things the body is continually trying to keep balanced is a long one and like many say...the struggle is real! So what am I doing that is assisting or undermining the balance my body is trying to maintain or return to?

Diagnosed to death: in July of 2013 the Journal of the American Medical Association (JAMA) published an article from researchers at the National Institute of Cancer that caused quite a stir, "Over diagnosis and Over treatment in Cancer: An Opportunity for Improvement." This should be a concern to all of us that get sucked into this loop since; carcinogens cause cancer and chemotherapy is carcinogenic, surgery and biopsies open cancer pockets in a barbaric (and potentially cancer spreading) manner, and radiation can actually cause cancer by messing up cellular DNA in an area.

Burning fat by controlling blood sugar:
lowering blood sugar is one of the simplest
strategies to trigger the fat burning process.
Lowering our blood sugar simply helps our body
recognize the need for another source of fuel, thus
triggering the release of energy substance from our
fat cells.

Burning fat with apple cider vinegar: excess
blood glucose is stored as fat and research has
shown that consuming 1 tablespoon of apple cider
vinegar in 8 oz. of water prior to mealtime,
reduced fasting blood glucose concentrations in
healthy adults at risk for type 2 diabetes.

The fat burning effect of food: surround
yourself with foods that take longer to digest (such
as raw vegetables, nuts and other unprocessed
foods). These foods trigger what is known as "the
thermic effect of food" and will burn more calories
throughout digestion vs. fast absorbing foods.

Fat burning tool chest for your kitchen:
oatmeal, eggs, apples, grapefruit, strawberries,
eggs, nuts, berries, broccoli, cauliflower, celery,

tomato, beans, quinoa, tuna (grilled fish), grilled chicken.

Burning fat through brain power: our body is one of the most powerful producers of personal designer drugs that we can ever hope for, and with the power our brain has, (with its signaling system of hormones and nerves throughout the body), I have no doubt it has the capability to increase metabolism, burn more fat and increase muscle gains, when we get a more vivid picture in our mind of what it is we are trying to do, while we're doing it.

The fat burning effect of compound exercises: if you want to increase the cardio and fat burning potential of your workout, do a lot of compound movements in the beginning of your routine and keep any of your individual muscle exercises at the end of your routine. This includes things such as biceps curl; triceps push downs, calf exercises, and leg extensions.

Pumping up the flab: fat with muscle pumped up under it actually can give a person a very healthy look and is one of the best short cuts for getting shaped up quickly! Rapid weight loss in the final weeks and days prior to an event will leave you looking saggy and unhealthy.

Sun Fitness: EVERYTHING on this planet would die without the sun. Getting too much exercise can be unhealthy; it's the same with the sun. Just like muscle, our skin conditions itself gradually to exposure.

Human Radiator: our body has powerful capabilities of heating and cooling itself, but we can do some things that make its job much easier and when we do this, it can put the energy saved toward giving us more energy for doing the things we have to do!

Tummy Flattening Effect of Fiber: one of the fastest ways to flatten our abdominal area is to eat a fiber rich diet, and I'm not referring to a cereal loaded diet, (most cereals spike blood sugar) but rather a diet that has lots of raw vegetables, beans, oatmeal, nuts and fruit in it. A diet rich in fiber helps prevent a buildup of waste in our waist!

We weigh too much because we...: the reason Americans on average weigh too much, is because we eat way too much! We really should become more need driven and a lot less pleasure driven with our fuel intake. This would take a huge burden off our food and our healthcare systems.

Pills, Guns and False Flags: false fear and confusion flags are for the purpose of diverting attention from the real thing, and one thing our government, media and pharmaceutical industry seem to all have in common, is their constant diversion of attention away from the underlying cause of the problems, and their appreciation for a good false flag to further their own agenda.

The human cell tower and its cellular language: our habits send out signals 24 hours a day, 7 days a week, 365 days a year to the several trillion cells in our body, whether for wellness or disease. We have the opportunity to speak health to the cells of our body through our healthy habits and the way we think and believe. The stronger and more positive we make these 3, the stronger the signal will be from our cell tower!

Gym of your future: your activities today are tomorrow's physical capability insurance! Whenever we have the opportunity at home, or work to do physical activity or manual labor, we should look at it as a muscle and fitness building opportunity. These are the real life exercises that help prevent injury when we attempt to do it tomorrow, next week and next year!

How negatives and injuries strengthen us: the positive things in life (and in exercise) look and feel great, but how we handle the negatives and recover from our injuries, plays a big part in building true strength, endurance and character!!

Personal designer drugs your body makes: your body not only produces drugs designed specifically for you and the bad things your body is fighting every day such as cancer, heart disease, stress etc. it also produces the chemicals that help increase energy, vitality and happiness! God designed something unmatchable when he designed our body's chemistry...

A fountain of violence they won't admit to: we have a conscious mind that is supposed to bother us, depress us and guide us to help us to make things better for ourselves and the ones we care about, so should we be throwing pills down our throat that tell our brains to chemically alter itself so as to not care or to feel differently about these things? If a person gets on S.S.R.I. drugs to help them suppress emotions, what happens if the conscious is suppressed...it's an emotion as well? It may feel good to a person to just not care, but how does it affect the ones that have to deal with this person? What happens if they suddenly get off the drug and their brain is as one on fire? When we have a massive amount of people on these drugs and an industry that is constantly pressing for even more expanded usage, what we will have left is a conscious suppressed generation of drug induced sociopaths that are like potential time bombs.

Controlling blood sugar with...: why would we rely on blood glucose control drugs that have many side affects, when we can control blood sugar spikes through food choices, activity and exercise, while at the same time reducing excess fatty deposits and cholesterol?

Childhood cancer and our early donor opportunity: we as parents are builders of the home our child's life resides in. This building process starts before conception, goes through the early stages of childhood and impacts their habits and decisions as a young adult and helps set the foundation for the next generation, (this is their body, they are our living legacy)!

Your child, your living legacy: our responsibility as parents should be to put a protective screen around our children by the lifestyle we show and teach them. One of the best insurance policies that we can leave with them, are the good habits that have shaped who they are and who they will become.

Pathways to suicide: there are pathways to

suicide that can become highways for someone that loses hope. We can only try to create pathways (for change and hope) around ourselves and the ones we care about. If you are someone that is contemplating ending it all, just don't do it, you still have a purpose in making the lives better for the ones you care about, in the ways only you can.

Are you at risk for breast cancer?: of course you are, if you have breast tissue (that is made up of glands, lobes, lobules, lymph vessels and lymph nodes). However, our body is constantly fixing things that are getting out of whack without us even knowing it. Each area of our body comes with its own system of cleansing, detoxification and repair mechanisms, so we should be looking for ways to strengthen that instead of constantly checking these areas to see if something is wrong with them.

Breast environment: mammograms expose the breast tissue and heart area to ionizing radiation. Quite simply, it is using the very thing to detect cancer that also happens to cause cancer. The painful compressions of the breast tissue come before the mammogram and since doctors are taught to NOT compress after a lump is found (because it can break the cancerous capsule), is not this a direct contradiction of proper procedure?

Breast cancer and hormone balance: hormones are messengers, and healthy lifestyle habits are what helps keep them balanced and from delivering weird messages to our corresponding, body parts or cells.

Breast cancer cell apoptosis, "nature's chemotherapy": healthy, consistent lifestyle habits not only can protect us from cancer, it can also shrink and eliminate the cancer. When we adapt healthy habits, our immune system and health can start immediately improving instead of getting slammed as most conventional (for profit) cancer treatment protocols do!

Holding your breath: temporarily holding your breath can give a slight surge in strength and help protect your back.

Cramps? Try pickle juice: pickle juice relieves cramps fast.

Pancreatic Cancer and Diabetes: If we can lighten the load on our pancreas, it just might help us avoid pancreatic cancer and diabetes. We can have small amounts of cancer in an organ such as the pancreas and never know it, but it can certainly affect its performance!

Flushing gallstones and healing our pancreas: there are ways to naturally flush our gallbladder don't let someone take yours without trying to flush it out first. Get on a high fiber diet and add in probiotics to help lower risk of gallstones and to relieve an overworked pancreas.

Reverse diabetes: don't get labeled, change your lifestyle to increase glucose uptake and lower the need for insulin.

HIV and the immune system: when we look at a compromised immune system and see how powerful a fully functional immune system is, we can better understand the healing and protective powers of this system that works 24-7-365 at protecting us!

Understanding the baby language of our parts: our aches and pains as well as the things that make us feel good, vibrant and refreshed are all trying to tell us something! Listening to your body and what it is trying to tell you is important, after all if you do not listen to your body who else will?

You are the parent of your body parts.

Endnote...

We have an awesome, beautiful, fun world that God has blessed us with and by staying mentally and physically healthy we can extract a much more fulfilling life and enjoy it more when we match our lifespan to our health span! We have the capability to do this without spending extra money; the tools for resistance, nutrition and other healthy lifestyle habits are all around us!

Example 1: there are ways to exercise that increase mobility and strength while at the same time increasing flexibility. When we teach multiple muscle groups to work together when we exercise, we match increased capabilities (in our exercise routine) to the life we want, whether it's sports, strength, manual labor capabilities, or simply increased mobility and independence.

Example 2: when we correct our lifestyle habits it gives our body the capability to produce the exact designer drugs our body needs to keep itself healthy and disease free.

Our immune system is like a laboratory and doctor that works 24 hours a day 365 days a year to fight disease and to keep things balanced and healthy!

I wish you the best in health and fitness

~ Wade Yoder

About the author

Wade Yoder has been in the health and fitness club business since 1991 and is a weekly health and fitness columnist for 5 Middle, Georgia newspapers with over 200 published articles since 2012.

He owns and operates Valley Athletic Club in Fort Valley, Georgia

Master Trainer certifications:

Fitness Trainer - Fitness Nutrition

Fitness Therapy - Strength and Conditioning - Senior Fitness – Youth Fitness

www.ingramcontent.com/pod-product-compliance
Lightning Source LLC
Chambersburg PA
CBHW062130280526
45788CB00001B/113